ADVANCE PRAISE ⌐○○ ○○ ○○○○ ┬ERRY

"Nick Terry has combined ancient wisdom, modern science, his own powerful life story and his actual breath practice to create a systematic guide to enhancing our lives through better breathing. Breath of Life is a revelatory book that will help readers unlock the secrets to living in balance and alignment."

–Dr. Nicholas Kardaras, Ph.D., LCSW, bestselling author of Glow Kids and former clinical professor at Stony Brook Medicine

BREATH OF LIFE

FINDING LONG-TERM RECOVERY WITH BREATHWORK AND STEPWORK

NICK TERRY TNT

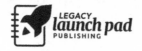

ISBN: 978-1-956955-87-3 (ebook)

ISBN: 978-1-956955-86-6 (paperback)

ISBN: 978-1-956955-85-9 (hardcover)

CONTENTS

Foreword   ix

PART 1
INTRODUCTION
Introduction   3
Beginner's Breathwork Routine   9

PART 2
NICK'S STORY
Chapter 1   15
Chapter 2   19
Chapter 3   30
Chapter 4   37
Chapter 5   42
Chapter 6   50
Chapter 7   56
Chapter 8   64
Chapter 9   69
Chapter 10   82
Chapter 11   90
Chapter 12   97

PART 3
EIGHT RECOVERY PRINCIPLES FOR
BREATHWORK WITH STEPWORK
Introduction   105
Testimonial: Marion's Story   109
1. Surrender   115
2. Clarity   120
3. Honesty   124
   Testimonial: Jeff's Story   129
4. Courage   139
5. Vulnerability   143

Testimonial: John's Story 149
6. Connection (Spiritual, Emotional, Physical) 153
7. Perseverance 158
8. Service and Spiritual Currency 164
   Testimonial: Travis's Story 171
   Conclusion 173

PART 4
BREATHWORK APPENDIX

Introduction 181
Breath Awareness 185
Cyclic Sighing 187
4-7-8 Breathing 189
Box Breathing 191
Three-Part Respiratory Breathing 193
Stimulating Breath 196
Tummo Breathing 198
Ujjayi Breathing 200
Alternate Nostril Breathing 202
Clarity Breathing and Breath of Life 204

Work with Nick Terry TNT 207
About the Author 211

I dedicate this book to my wife, Paulina TNT, for motivating me to write my story and constantly reminding me that I am overqualified. To my daughters, Coco and Steisha, for bringing so much light and joy into my life. To all those who have carried a message of recovery and showed me the way to living a happy, joyous and free life.

And finally, to all of those who haven't found peace, joy or freedom from active addiction, depression, anxiety, grief or trauma—my deepest intention is that this book can be as helpful to you as possible.

FOREWORD

Everything in life starts with the breath: the literal source of life for all humans, though it is so often neglected or forgotten. Indeed, people will forget to breathe during times of high stress, will have to "catch their breath" when exerting themselves or will breathe shallowly when not mindful or in the present moment. In my native Greek, *pneuma*, the word for breath, also translates to the literal word for "spirit" or "soul"—that's how inextricably linked our breathing is to our very essence.

Indeed, many survivalists are keenly aware of the 3-3-30 rule: a human can only survive three minutes without air, three days without water and 30 days without food (generally speaking, though of course there are outliers). Thus, among food, water and air, breathing is the most fundamental and necessary of all biological functions.

Yet, unlike eating, it's also an autonomic function; we breathe without even having to do anything or think about it. It just happens: while we sleep, while we're driving and while we run to catch a bus. But even though it's an autonomic function, somehow we modern humans have found a way to complicate things, mucking up this most natural of processes.

Because our breathing is tied to our autonomic nervous system, encompassing both the sympathetic nervous system (the fight or flight response) and parasympathetic nervous system (the resting state), breathing both *reflects* our nervous state (or our emotional state) and can also act as a cue to help *regulate* or even *cause* emotional or nervous states. Unfortunately, the post-industrial, 21st century world has created conditions wherein we're almost always in a state of fight or flight, also known as HPA activation (an activation of our hypothalamus-pituitary-adrenal axis). HPA activation is a feedback loop that spikes our adrenaline so that we can have the fuel to run or fight if we perceive a threat. The HPA axis does this by pumping oxygen from our hearts into our bloodstream, and by pumping air into our lungs to maximize our capacity for an impending, life-sustaining event.

But here's the rub: in the natural world of our ancestors, the HPA response was very time-limited and specific to actual threats, such as a lion in the high grass or a crocodile coming out of the water. Once the threat went away, our adrenal thermostat—and our breathing—would go back to normal. But that's not the case today. Today, we live in a high-adrenaline, activated world of sensory overload. Our adrenal thermostats are on perpetual high alert, and we're breathing as if we're always in danger. It's the modern plague of high anxiety, which from a breathing standpoint translates into shallow, rapid breaths or even an unconscious holding of one's breath. We literally "forget" to breathe.

As a psychologist who has run treatment programs all over the world, I've worked with clients who are struggling with all manner of psychiatric distresses, including depression, anxiety and addiction. Oftentimes, they seek answers outside of themselves through medications, therapists, psychiatrists, life coaches, shamans and religious gurus, all of which can be beneficial. Still, what so often gets neglected is the power of breathing: the power of breath techniques to re-tune our frequency towards health, healing and wholeness. That's where my dear friend Nick Terry comes in.

I've known Nick for many years as a dedicated and compassionate man in recovery. He is not only what we might call a "seeker" but a healer as well. I first got to know Nick as someone of the utmost integrity who committed himself to helping others find their true path and transform. At first, his toolbox consisted of the 12 Steps and life coaching techniques —wonderful and potentially life-saving tools which certainly helped me immensely on my healing path.

But somewhere on Nick's journey, as he describes in this beautiful and practical book, he discovered the magic and power of breath, namely the secrets and transformative potential of breathwork. We know from clinical research that techniques like meditation can be amazingly effective for stress, depression and anxiety. We can now consider breathwork in that same hallowed category, only perhaps it is even more practical, easier to use and with more exciting potential. We see this in practitioners like Wim Hof, who can do seemingly miraculous things with the mastery of his breath, whether it's changing his core body temperature as he swims under polar ice caps, or fortifying his immune system to the point that it rejects botulism injected in his body. His feats are legendary.

As a teen, I studied martial arts with Sensei Hidy Ochiai, with whom I learned not only the power of deep Sanchin breathing, but also the technique of "breath mirroring" one's opponent in a sparring match. When you mirror your opponent's breath, you can essentially inhabit their emotional and psychic state, thus anticipating their next move. Years later, as a therapist, I found that when I used breath mirroring with clients, it unlocked the door to deep empathy and understanding, almost like the breath version of the Vulcan mind meld.

With this book, Nick Terry has given us all a wonderful gift. He has taken ancient wisdom, modern science, his own powerful life story and his actual breath practice, and created a book that takes a systematic look at how a person may learn to master their breathing in order to enhance their lives.

This is an amazing and revelatory book which will help readers unlock the secret to living a life of balance and alignment, with a sense of true purpose that satisfies their souls—and I encourage them to breathe it all in.

–*Dr. Nicholas Kardaras, Ph.D., LCSW,*
bestselling author of *Glow Kids* and former
clinical professor at Stony Brook Medicine

PART 1

INTRODUCTION

INTRODUCTION

I was first introduced to breathwork at a Quepasana retreat on the beautiful island of Maui. It was a meditation course that took 10 days and instructed participants to observe noble silence on a pristine, oceanfront property on the southernmost tip of Makena Maui. The daily schedule consisted of six hours of sitting meditation, four hours of yin yoga, breathwork practice and inspired vegan cuisine. I was four years sober, but the course was still fairly advanced for me considering that my meditation practice at the time consisted of 10 to 15-minute-long sessions with a guided app (assuming I was meditating at all, which I often wasn't).

On the retreat, I was introduced to an unfamiliar breathing style. I didn't get to ask questions about it since I had to remain silent (though one of the teachers said the techniques were a way of "getting high on your own supply"). Several weeks later, I learned that the technique was made famous as the eponymous Wim Hof Method, even though it actually dates back thousands of years and is also known as Tibetan Tummo breathing.

This technique felt awkward to me at first and triggered feelings of anxiety. At times it almost felt like I was suffocating, but I tried to trust the process and stick with it. At the beginning, I was able to hold my breath for one minute. After a few rounds, it was 90 seconds—and at my longest, I was able to hold my breath for around two minutes.

I was fascinated by this. I had never been able to hold my breath for that long, especially without any oxygen in my lungs. I imagined I was becoming more oxygenated, but more importantly, every time I did the breath practice, I felt completely alive, focused and alert. I was consciously connected and firing on all cylinders.

When the 10 days were over, I left with a new perspective. In the most poetic sense, it felt like some part of me had died, yet at the same time, I came to believe death didn't even exist. All of the participants left the course with deeper and richer meditation and breathing practices, including myself.

Most people aren't aware of their breathing because it happens unconsciously. After nine years of sobriety, and having worked in the field of mental health and substance abuse treatment for the last eight years, I can tell you that about 80 percent of people who struggle with addiction also report having some type of anxiety or depression (and usually both). What I've learned working in addiction recovery and through my research into breathwork over the last few years is that unprocessed grief and trauma present as anxiety, panic and depression. Often, all three are occurring simultaneously.

In my own experiences with recovery, I saw people who didn't want to do 12-step programs at all, or who would abandon the program around the time they started to do a fourth step inventory. It was a seemingly universal experience, something that almost any long-term member of the 12-step community can attest to—and there are a million different reasons why people won't complete that fourth step.

My theory is that when we start attending any recovery-based program, we are usually pretty broken and willing to change, or else we wouldn't be there in the first place. What I've seen over and over is that our willingness starts to dwindle the longer we maintain abstinence. What starts as a commitment to long-term sobriety turns into, "Do I *have* to attend a meeting every day?" This usually occurs somewhere between Day 30 and Day 120. Interestingly, it also tends to correlate with the beginning of some kind of personal inventory process, regardless of the program.

People give many explanations for why they stop attending support groups, whether it's the other members of the group, the dogmatic and archaic nature of the literature, or the stigma of identifying as an addict or alcoholic. But at the core of this avoidance is fear, anxiety, depression, unprocessed grief and unconscious trauma-response patterns. The 12-step recovery community and others like it are "spiritual programs," meaning they talk about God, prayer and spiritual awakenings. Though they often include some kind of meditation practice, one thing missing from this equation is breathwork.

Needless to say, the act of breathing is deeply connected to a sense of inner peace and spirituality across countless different cultures and religions. Given that universality, it is my belief that a return to the breath is the missing piece of addiction recovery in the West.

I still love AA to this day: I attend several meetings a week, I regularly connect with my sponsor and volunteer to sponsor newcomers who need guidance. But what's been abundantly clear to me over the years is that we need something new. We need a new program—a "breath of fresh air," if you will—or at least something non-dogmatic to help people stay tethered to recovery. What I've tried to develop in this book is a guide, modeled from the Big Book, to what the recovery world has been missing: breathwork.

This book is set up in several parts.

Part I encompasses the foreword, this introduction and a sample breathwork routine that anyone can get started using right away. In Part II, I tell my own full story of recovery from childhood to the present, explaining the obstacles I faced, what led me to addiction and how I was able to overcome it through 12 Steps and breathwork. Part III gives a series of updated principles of stepwork and breathwork, along with testimonials and personal stories from other recovering addicts who have had great success putting these techniques into practice. Finally, Part IV is a breathwork appendix with a list of breathwork terms, routines and other exercises to help readers start their own practices.

For anyone who hasn't found the success they were looking for in 12-Step recovery, or who has been in and out of the rooms over the years (like I was for half a decade), this book is for you. By using breathwork, anyone can enhance, expand and further develop their spiritual life to maximize their usefulness to others and realize their deepest potential in this present moment. This approach is compatible with 12-Step teachings, though following AA to the letter isn't required for you to still get the benefits. In addition to helping with substance abuse challenges, the methods I describe here can also help with mental health challenges such as anxiety and depression, or compulsive behaviors like digital addiction, excessive screen time, gambling, sex, pornography, and codependency.

In my life, the results of breathwork speak for themselves. With my new sense of inner calm, I am now married to my best friend, which is a miracle: two years ago, I was convinced I "just didn't know how to do relationships." Without breathwork, I would have never been able to write this book, develop a new recovery program or meet my life partner. It has allowed me to tap into my creativity and focus with previously unrealized clarity and passion. I currently own and operate a residential mental health and substance abuse treatment center called Honu House Hawaii, on the Kona side of the beautiful Big Island. We do daily breathwork, cold plunges, hyperbaric oxygen chamber sessions, recovery groups, holistic healing, horticulture and other amazing healing modalities. All of this happened in the last 13 months—along with meeting Wim Hof to hike the Spanish Pyrenees and interview him in an ice bath, while we freestyle-rapped and he beatboxed (WTF, I know).

Physically, I'm in the best shape of my life. I do CrossFit five days a week and surf every day (at least, whenever there are waves). Before adopting these new practices, I was constantly caught up in discord, arguments and reactive engagements that dominated my thoughts all the time—but not anymore. My hope is that this book can give the same transformation to anyone who reads it.

–Nick Terry, 2023

BEGINNER'S BREATHWORK ROUTINE

Ever since I learned about breathwork, I've been getting "high on my own supply" while also creating and trying other structured breath practices daily. I've also started teaching these methods, patterns and routines to clients at my residential treatment center as well as to private clients, and the results have been magnificent.

To get started helping anyone who wants to begin with breathwork, I've included my own daily routine here. I invite you to use it and make it your own, though it's worth mentioning a few quick safety notes: never do breathwork while driving and never do breathwork alone while submerged in any body of water (even if it's just in a shallow pool or tub). Now, on to the exercise:

1. Wake up early in the morning (I usually wake up around 4:30 am). There may be some worry and fear lingering in your mind as you begin to plan and design your day. This is normal; the breathwork will help it evaporate.

2. Make a cup of hot tea with lemon and find a comfortable place to sit or lie down. Personally, I like to go sit on my lanai under the stars.

3. Begin breathing deeply into the bottom of your belly and then your chest. Allow yourself to fully expand before exhaling and letting it all go—do all of this in one breath. The emphasis is on inhalation: big into the belly, up to the chest and a soft exhale instead of a forceful outbreath. For rhythm, think of breathing in for two and letting go for one: *belly, chest, let go; belly, chest, let go,* or *in-in-out, in-in-out.*

4. Repeat this process for 35 breaths. On the 35th, completely exhale and hold for as long as it feels comfortable (usually anywhere between 45 and 90 seconds). It's not a contest, so only do what feels right for you.

5. Repeat this entire process at least four times and for up to seven rounds every morning.

6. As your system becomes completely oxygenated through your rounds of breathing, try to shift your state of consciousness. Sit quietly in meditation for five to 15 minutes. I recommend a minimum of five minutes, but do whatever feels best, remembering that you can develop a longer practice over time.

7. After your breathwork, write down three things you are grateful for, three things you can do to make that day amazing and a long list of "I am" affirmations. For example: "I am an amazing author. I am successful. I am loved. I am a great father or mother. I am connected. I am a healer. I am healing. I am married. I am loved." Write down your affirmations in the present tense, even if you

haven't accomplished them yet. At the end of the day before bed, review your day and see if you accomplished the three things you wrote down to make your day great. Write down one thing you could have done better.

The next part of the routine is completing the 4-7-8 breathing. This can be done anytime, and I recommend doing it several times, around midday, afternoon and evening. It is also very simple:

1. Breathe in deeply through your nose for four seconds, expanding your rib cage.
2. Hold your breath for seven seconds.
3. Release your breath slowly out your mouth for eight seconds, making a long *haaa* sound.
4. Repeat this pattern for five to 10 rounds.

I do all of the above every day, and it is my natural antidepressant medication—I also have a guided breathwork track you can access using this barcode:

Throughout your day, you may notice some difficult feelings come up: old patterns, trauma responses, anger, fear, jealousy, resentment and life challenges. As you do this practice, remind yourself to breathe into them. For example, if you feel some discomfort arise, immediately take a slow, deep breath in for four seconds through the nose, hold it for seven seconds and then slowly exhale for eight seconds. You can repeat this pattern for three to four rounds, and it works like magic to alleviate stress. Whenever I do public speaking, I use the same pattern and the nervousness slips away.

All throughout your day, remember to constantly breathe in slower through the nose, holding and gently letting go. You can do it while driving in traffic, while at work, when writing and reading or any other time you remember to do these exercises.

I've been practicing daily breathwork for the last four years, and the results have been amazing. The recovery community often puts emphasis on meditation, and while meditation is a powerful technique, I find that it can be a little too advanced for most people in early recovery. It wasn't until I had a daily breathwork practice that I really experienced the benefits of meditation, which is why I recommend first focusing on your breathing.

Even before you get very far into this book, try jumping into these breathing routines right away—try them right now. Track your results and write out your gratitude lists. If you get nothing else from this book besides the breathwork routine outlined above, you will still make a tremendous difference in your life.

PART 2

NICK'S STORY

CHAPTER ONE

I was born June 3, 1979 in Eugene, Oregon when my mother was 18 and my dad was 20. Though they were married at the time, my mother divorced my dad before my first birthday because of his dishonesty and infidelity. According to her, there were several instances of betrayal and unfaithfulness, and she decided to divorce when she came home early from a trip and found that all their wedding and baby pictures had been removed from the walls and hidden out of sight to accommodate whoever his guests were. According to my grandmother, my mother became a little more wild and adventurous after her marriage ended. Who could blame her? She was young, beautiful and free from a toxic relationship.

When I was five years old, my mom and I left Oregon for the big city of Seattle, Washington—along with her boyfriend Marty and their rock and roll band. My earliest memories are of booze-fueled parties that went late into the night. It was the early 1980s and sex, drugs and rock and roll were part of the culture. Meanwhile, I was right in the middle of it.

Though it's difficult to remember everything from my

childhood exactly, I do remember falling asleep on the floor and waking up to strangers lying on the couch with empty bottles of alcohol scattered around. One morning when I was around seven years old, I saw a plate by the couch with a short, cut-up straw on it, along with some white, powdery residue. I stuck my finger in to taste it and it was bitter. I thought it was medicine, though of course later in life I realized it was cocaine.

Over the course of my childhood, my mom and her friends used cocaine, alcohol and marijuana. Later on, they advanced to crystal meth and heroin, and my mom developed a significant addiction as well as a depression that lasted throughout her life. As I grew up, nobody ever sat me down and explicitly told me, *Nick, we don't talk about this with other people—don't tell anybody at school what's happening at home!* Even so, it was something I learned to hide intuitively; it was an unspoken expectation. From a young age, instead of being open, honest and transparent, I started closing myself off, being dishonest and secretive. It was the beginning of a pattern. Though I didn't realize it at the time, I also believe it's when my spiritual malady started to develop.

Because I still wanted to connect with other kids and tell them things about me and my life, I started making up stories I could say out loud. When I was eight years old, my mom, her new husband Rob and I lived on Bainbridge Island, a ferry ride across the Puget Sound from downtown Seattle. My real dad was not around; he was living in Eugene at the time. Like my mom, he has also struggled with a lifetime of substance abuse and mental health challenges.

In those days, I spent a lot of time playing basketball and I'd gotten pretty good. One day, I was on the court at my elementary school when I told the other kids that my dad was Tom Chambers. Tom Chambers was a 6'10" professional basketball player on the Seattle Supersonics, and one of the only white guys on the team. I was a huge fan.

"Tom Chambers is not your dad," one of the kids said. "If your dad is an NBA basketball player, why do you guys live in that little apartment?" Despite their obvious objections, I fully committed to the lie and refused to let it go—to the point where the teacher had to intervene.

"Nick says his dad is Tom Chambers. Is that true?" one of the kids asked Miss White, our teacher.

"Now, Nick," Miss White said carefully, "Tom Chambers is not your dad." I started crying.

"He is my dad; he is my dad!" I insisted, hyperventilating.

I let it go for a while, but later at a parent-teacher conference, my mom came in with her husband and some of the kids approached them.

"Is Tom Chambers really Nick's dad?" the kids asked her. She looked puzzled—I don't think she even knew who Tom Chambers was at the time.

"Nick's dad lives in Eugene," she said.

On top of lying about who my dad was, I lied to kids about how many video games I had and how rich my family was. I lied about how many pairs of shoes I owned and about my basketball, baseball and football card collections. Very quickly, lying became a part of who I was—and so did stealing things on a regular basis.

When I was in preschool and kindergarten, my crimes began to escalate. On a school field trip, my class was walking around a store when I took a pack of gum off the shelf and slipped it into my pocket. I wasn't sure why I did it, and after we left the store and were far enough away, I pulled the packet out and showed the teacher what had happened, acting like it was an accident.

"Uh-oh," my teacher replied. "You'll have to be more

careful next time!" Seeing that there were no consequences, I started shoplifting more and more, for no real reason. Just like I'd done the first time, whenever I was in a store, I would slip things like gum or candy in my pocket and walk out without paying for them, daring someone to notice. Nobody ever stopped me, and I never got in trouble for it.

Later on, my mom started dating Jack, a rock musician. We were staying at his apartment when I decided to search through one of his cabinets. After rummaging around, I found $20— which was a lot of money at the time. *Lucky me,* I thought. I put the money in my pocket and kept it there for a couple of days, not knowing what else to do with it. A few nights later, I was with my mom at the restaurant where she worked. We were sitting in the hostess area up front, and I decided to put the $20 on the ground and pretend like I'd just found it.

"Oh my gosh, Mom, look!" I said. "I just found $20 on the ground!" She didn't have a lot of money at the time, so she was excited too, and it felt good to share that moment with her. I thought nothing of it and figured I had covered my tracks— until a few months later, her boyfriend started hunting for the money he'd lost.

Of course, I played dumb and acted like I had no clue what he was talking about.

CHAPTER TWO

A year or so later, my mom married a guy named Rob, who proposed after just a few weeks of dating. Rob was a dishwasher at a local restaurant by day and a drummer by night, while my mom worked as a waitress. I don't remember much from that season of my childhood, but I do remember being home alone a lot when I was seven and eight years old, left to eat Cheetos and candy and watch television until I fell asleep. I loved the sitcoms: *Three's Company, Gilligan's Island, The A-Team, Growing Pains, Mr. Belvedere, Different Strokes* and *The Golden Girls*, to name a few. When I could stay up late enough, sometimes WWF, NWA or GLOW, the Gorgeous Ladies of Wrestling, would come on, and I fell in love with those shows as well. All of them offered me a first real escape from reality, long before marijuana and alcohol.

Gradually, the fear of being alone was replaced by an excitement for the sense of comfort and connection I would find while watching those shows.

One night, my mom and Rob were at a house party, and I must have fallen asleep in the back of our old black Volkswagen

Beetle because I woke up and nobody was there. It was cold, dark and I was extremely scared. I got out of the car and yelled for them but quickly realized I had no clue which house they were in, and I knew they couldn't hear me. As quickly as I had jumped out of the car, I jumped back in and lay down in the backseat again. Absolutely terrified, I cried myself back to sleep. Though the details are hard to remember, and they must have come back to the car at some point, what I do remember from that time is feeling separate and different, alone and afraid.

When I was nine or 10 years old, my mom got a job as a waitress at the Columbia Tower Club Restaurant in downtown Seattle, a 45-minute ferry ride from where we lived on Bainbridge Island. At that time, she and Rob were growing apart for many reasons, one of which was his drug and alcohol addiction. While working her new job, my mom met a fellow waiter named Tom, and it was love at first sight. Although she was married, my mom and Tom quickly started developing a relationship. Within a few months, we had moved off Bainbridge Island and into a small two-bedroom home with Tom in Queen Anne Hill. Soon after, my mom finalized her divorce. Our life was like that, I was learning; one day we were in one place, the next day we were gone.

Tom was about five years younger than my mom and only 12 years older than I was. We got along pretty well, and I came to love living in Queen Anne Hill. I made many friends at the local recreation center, where I started to develop my lifelong love of basketball, and I got my first job as a paperboy delivering *The Seattle Times*. In the sixth grade, I got a job as a deli clerk at Ken's Market, and used my earnings to help out with the groceries at home—and to buy candy and snacks to share at school. As the new kid in town, I was popular with the girls at school, and soon came to love my new life—but things changed when my mom and Tom started to experiment with heroin.

Their addictions progressed throughout the three years they dated, and our life got worse and worse—but things came to a head when Tom's friend Dillon overdosed in our living room. Dillon was a colleague of his from work. He seemed like a nice man, and I'd even met his wife. Then one day, he was lying lifeless on our kitchen floor and my mom was screaming at me to call the paramedics. Seeing my mom come unhinged, I ran to the phone and called 911 as she directed me from the background.

"Why is he on the ground seizing up?" the dispatcher asked me.

"I don't know," I replied, "he just fell down and isn't responding."

"He had a heroin overdose," my mom shouted in the background. "Just get the fucking ambulance here as soon as possible!"

"Did she say he had a heroin overdose?" the dispatcher asked.

"Yes, that's what she said," I replied. "Please hurry."

Though Dillon survived, the experience shook everyone involved, and I started putting things together that I hadn't before. I remembered some men who used to stop by our house from time to time to use our telephone, who I now realized were heroin dealers. I also remembered a few times Tom had to pawn my baseball and basketball cards to get money; on another occasion, it was my stereo. All along, he'd needed the money for drugs.

As he came to grips with what had happened, Tom told my mom that he needed to try to get sober, and that they should do it together. She agreed, and they got on methadone, but trying to get off heroin was making things increasingly unstable between them. Eventually, it was decided that I'd spend the ninth grade with my dad and his wife Lauren in Oregon. My dad had struggled with drug addiction throughout my life as well, but at that time he was stable. I knew that things must have been pretty bad for my mom to have even considered letting me go. I could tell it broke her heart, even if it was the best option under the circumstances.

I didn't know my dad very well, since I'd only spent summer vacations, Christmas breaks and a handful of visits to Seattle with him. I didn't trust or respect him much. But for a year in Eugene, things went pretty well. I was the new kid on campus, and again I made fast friends. I even made the freshman basketball team, as tryouts were being held the exact same day I started at Sheldon High. Though I lacked structure, discipline and good study habits, I passed my classes at the beginning of freshman year.

At the end of the year, my mom decided to leave Tom and move to Eugene to be closer to me and the rest of her family. It would also be a fresh start, away from heroin and methadone. Tom went to stay in a sober living in Seattle, and I moved out of my dad's house to move into an apartment with my mom. At the time, I had no clue that she was going through one of the hardest detox processes imaginable. She was going cold turkey off her methadone maintenance program, and didn't get a single night of rest for a month. When I found out, I was heart-broken. I had been ridiculing her for always misplacing the car keys, and being frazzled and absentminded, not knowing there were reasons for her shortcomings. Unfortunately, after my mom finally finished detoxing, she hooked up with a guy named Phil who had zero interest in sobriety.

Phil was a marijuana grower and crystal meth addict from the moment we met him, and it was also clear that he was a gangster of some kind. He lived a dangerous life, and soon my mom joined him, becoming a daily crystal meth user herself. As things got more dangerous at my mom's house, I spent more time with my dad again. Since he was working a program, he would occasionally take me with him to AA meetings, hoping that some of it would rub off. At the time, all I saw was a bunch of losers smoking cigarettes in church basements and complaining about their lives. My dad had been in AA his whole life, even when he was drinking and doing drugs, so I wasn't convinced that it worked at all.

As Phil and my mom kept dating, I made friends with Phil's son Jake, and he became like a brother to me. We were both in the 10th grade and had similar interests: primarily partying, smoking weed and listening to and making our own rap music. Everyone in our social sphere looked up to Phil; he always had a wad of cash on him and he owned a '51 Chevy lowrider. He was a Chicano gangster from Los Angeles with a Rasta mystique about him. Unfortunately, when Phil did drugs, he became a lot less cool and a lot more unpredictable.

As Phil yelled and got violent more often, my mom became desperate for a way out. She had stayed in touch with Tom in Seattle, who had succeeded in getting a month or two sober and wanted to reconnect with us. To my knowledge, he had no idea my mom was already deep in another relationship.

Regardless, my mom talked to my grandma about our situation, and she agreed that we needed a change.

"You need to get away from Phil as fast as you can," my grandmother said. "Even if you don't have the money, I'm happy to help." Since staying with Phil was a terrible option, the plan was for my mom to meet Tom in Portland, halfway between Eugene and Seattle, to talk about getting back together and what that would mean for their future. In the meantime, my grandma would give Tom money for an apartment in Seattle that was big enough for the three of us.

When the big day came to escape Phil and meet Tom in Portland, my mom never showed up. She had been on a crystal meth binge that made her lose track of time, keeping her stuck in Eugene. After realizing my mom wasn't coming, Tom went back to Seattle, used the rent money my grandma had given him to buy heroin and died of an overdose that night. My mom was beside herself when she heard the news, blaming herself for his death and burying herself in shame and regret. Her addiction issues had already been bad, but Tom's death made them so much worse.

My parents' turbulent relationships meant I spent my childhood bouncing back and forth between houses, landing wherever the grown-ups were relatively less dangerous. Things took another turn when my dad's brother died from HIV/AIDS when I was 15, sending my dad into a spiral that led him to another relapse. With chaos and tragedy all around me, I looked for any escape I could. Often, it was sneaking off with Jake to smoke weed and drink, but it also meant playing a lot of basketball, the only thing I really liked about school. During those years when I was moving and transferring schools almost constantly, at least I had basketball as a constant stress reliever.

Both my mom and dad were too busy battling their own demons to pay attention to me or make sure I was keeping up with my schoolwork. As a result, I did almost none of it. Unfortunately, it turned out that you needed to earn at least a C-average to stay on the basketball team, so even though I had the skills to pass tryouts, I didn't have the GPA—and I was kicked off the team in 10th grade. With my only healthy outlet now gone, I didn't improve my grades. Instead, I doubled down on living a stoner lifestyle, living only for the moment, with no thoughts about the future.

One day when I was 16 years old, I was walking the halls of my school, half-baked, when two girls approached me.

"Hey Nick," they murmured with a grin. "Do you think you could sell us some weed?" Though nobody had asked me that before, it made sense that they would—after all, I looked like a stoner. Though I had some weed in my pocket, I hadn't been planning on selling any of it.

"Sorry, girls," I replied. "I've got a little for me but not enough to sell."

"Aw, please?" one of the girls asked. "Let us see it at least!" I discreetly pulled the baggie out of my pocket to show them before putting it away.

"That's plenty!" they replied. "We barely want any, just enough for a joint. We can give you $10?" Since I was already stoned, the situation was getting awkward, and I had no cash for McDonald's later, I finally agreed to sell them a little bit of my stash—and when school was out, I went to the corner to get a McChicken, fries and a drink. *Now this is the good life,* I thought.

I was still high and a little hungry when I got home so I started making myself a peanut butter and jelly sandwich. Suddenly, I was interrupted by a knock on the door. I opened it to reveal Officer Fitzpatrick, my school's police liaison, who pushed his way in without an invitation.

"Hey Nick," he said. "I caught a couple students smoking marijuana today. I asked them where they got it from and they told me your name. Got anything to say about that?" I shrugged and shook my head no. "It's not a big deal," he said casually. "It's just a lil' weed. I won't arrest you if you tell me you sold it to them."

Though I was far from a drug dealer at the time—just a garden variety stoner—I knew enough from Phil and the other criminals who populated my life not to tell on myself. For some reason though, that didn't stop me from doing it anyway.

"I gave them the weed," I said with a sense of relief. "I don't normally sell it; it was just my personal stash." Officer Fitzpatrick nodded.

"Don't worry," he said. "Again, it's just a little pot, so I'm not going to arrest you. I'll just need you to sign a few documents and I'll be on my way." I had always heard that the truth would set you free—but I soon learned that didn't apply when you were talking to the police.

After telling the truth, I was swiftly expelled from school for the distribution of a controlled substance within a thousand feet of school property, a Class B felony. Since I'd already gone through so many schools, my mom enrolled me in an alternative high school full of pregnant girls smoking cigarettes and kids who were only attending because they'd brought weapons to the schools *they'd* been kicked out of. From then on, instead of hanging out with the wrong crowd, I *was* the wrong crowd, and any hope I'd ever had of playing basketball was now gone for good. In total, I attended 14 schools in 11 years.

The subjects at the Opportunity Center were things like "movies" and "walking," and there was almost no attempt to teach us anything interesting. Instead, it was just a holding place for misfits, burnouts and future criminals. Everything was so easy that it was almost insulting, and it seemed like if I stayed there, I would be increasing my chances of turning into a criminal myself. Though I never got kicked out, after only a month or so I stopped attending completely—and nobody stopped me.

As part of the sentencing conditions of my felony I had attend adolescent drug treatment, but I did everything I could to defy the rules. Things were going well for a while, and I considered myself resourceful for passing drug tests by using other people's urine. I was successfully playing the system, and through some legal loophole, I didn't have to continue with the program as an adult. I didn't graduate or get a certificate, but when I turned 18, I quit going—and started hanging out with other druggies and petty criminals like me.

When I was 18, I found a new crew in a kind of rap group and gang called the Black Mobb Family, who let me join even though I was an 18-year-old white boy. We were part of a local culture of pimps and rappers, and we sold drugs and hung out with prostitutes. The more time I spent in the gang, the more I started to think of myself as a gangster—and before long, I was selling cocaine and living a criminal lifestyle, all while trying to launch a rap career like everyone else around me.

Shortly after I'd started down that path, I was hanging out at a house with Shab Won, a friend of mine in the Black Mobb Family. I had a few small bags of cocaine in my pocket. Shab had somehow borrowed a 20-gauge shotgun from my mom's boyfriend Phil, and he was horsing around with it in the backyard. While he was playing with it, the gun went off—*BOOM!* Fortunately, it had been pointed at the ground and no one got hurt, but it was the loudest thing I'd ever heard, and it wasn't long before the cops showed up.

We were still sitting obliviously in the backyard when we heard the telltale sirens closing in. In a flash, Shab jumped out of his chair and ran inside, slamming the door behind him and leaving me outside as cops swarmed the backyard with guns pointed at me.

"Freeze!" they shouted. "Get your hands up!" I was terrified and dropped to my knees, doing exactly as they said. A moment later, one of the officers came up to pat me down and found the three bags of cocaine in my pocket that I'd forgotten about—*just* after I'd finally gotten off probation from my adolescent charges.

"You're under arrest, son," the cop growled, putting me in handcuffs. From lying, shoplifting and getting busted for selling a little weed, I had finally graduated to my first, real adult drug charge: cocaine possession. Though I was supposed to go to court for that, I had no intention of sticking around to find out what would happen to me if I did. Instead, I decided to skip town to California with a girlfriend of mine, where she started making money doing sex work. I was constantly drinking and smoking weed to escape my internal dialogue about my life, but nevertheless, there I was—living it.

After just two months in the Bay Area, a friend and I were pulled over by the police for questioning. They wanted to know about our connection to a friend of ours, who was a sex worker. As they interrogated us, it was never clear what they were accusing us of or what they were investigating, and I tried to say as little as possible. They were about to let me go when they ran my ID, found out about my outstanding warrant in Oregon and decided to throw me in county jail instead.

Since my crime was a felony that had happened in Oregon, I was going to be extradited from California by a company called Transcorp America, which transported prisoners across state lines. I spent 30 days in Martinez County Jail in Richmond, California. Martinez is one of the worst jails in the state, with real gangsters and violent criminals—and then there was me, 18 years old and 160 pounds, soaking wet. Although I was terrified, I ended up getting along with my cellmate and tried to pass the days playing handball, watching TV, playing cards and reading. After 30 days, they read my name over the intercom.

"Terry, Nick," a voice called out. "Roll up your stuff, it's time to go." Since I wasn't that far from where I needed to go in Oregon, I assumed the drive would take 10 hours or so. Unfortunately, getting me from California to Oregon efficiently was not a top priority for the van's driver, and the itinerary was subject to change at a moment's notice. In all, I spent *eight days* driving across the country in the back of that van with other hardcore criminals before I finally made it to Oregon. When I arrived, I finally found out what the California cops were investigating me for: sex trafficking. Though I was shocked and had nothing to do with what I was accused of, I knew that didn't matter. If I got convicted, I would get 100 months in prison—and on top of that, I'd be labeled a sex offender for the rest of my life.

My grandfather hired a lawyer who advised me what to say and what not to say, all while I considered the possibility of serious prison time. When the time came to hear my case, by some stroke of incredible luck, the prosecution didn't have enough evidence to make their charges stick. Instead, the charges were lowered, then dropped altogether. After that narrow escape, I had a court appointment to deal with my outstanding cocaine possession charge—but I had other plans.

I have to get away from all this, I thought, imagining a new start for myself, far from all the drugs and criminals surrounding me. *If I can go far away, I know I can make a fresh start and things will get better.* Fortunately, an opportunity came through my cousin Bill, who was born and raised on Maui and had moved back to Eugene to go to college at the University of Oregon. Although we'd partied a lot together, he was always able to manage his lifestyle effectively, and he'd even earned high marks in all of his college classes.

Bill and I were like brothers, and he knew what kind of path I was on. He accepted all of my collect calls from jail and he took care of me financially when I needed help. Finally, while he was on Christmas break, he offered to take me with him to Hawaii in 1998—and like that, I left the Pacific Northwest for Maui when I was 19 years old.

CHAPTER THREE

When I got to Maui, nobody knew who I was or where I came from. It was the same feeling I'd had so many times before when I was transferring between schools, eager to tell new stories and reinvent myself—only this time, I was going to do things differently. I still wasn't planning on telling anyone the truth, of course, and I would leave out as much as I could about my family history and my legal troubles. Instead, I would try to get a basic job and live a normal life, leaving all my worries behind me.

After a few interviews, I got a job as a busser at a local restaurant and gradually worked my way up to being a waiter, which paid a little better. The change in scenery brightened my spirits, and I made friends with some of the people I worked with in the restaurant. Though I was mostly free from the kinds of violent criminals I'd known in Washington and Oregon, people in restaurants still liked to party, and I quickly got absorbed into the lifestyle.

Before, I just liked to drink and smoke weed. But now I was

partying every night after my shifts, advancing to harder drugs like Molly and cocaine. And as much fun as I was having meeting new people and living it up on the island, all the drugs and drinking were taking a toll on my body and my bank account. I made good money as a waiter, but anything extra went to getting high, and I had little left over. After spinning in that same cycle for five years, my energy levels were dropping, and it was hard to keep up at work.

Now I was starting to worry about myself and my future again. Just like when I'd first arrived in Maui, I told myself I needed a break from the people and the lifestyle surrounding me or else something bad would happen. Once again, maybe all I needed was a change in location.

If I can get away from all this, I can get back on the right track, I thought to myself. *I'll go back to Oregon and set everything straight. I'll finally deal with my legal troubles, and I'll explain that I only left the state to sober up and live a more upstanding life. They'll understand.*

Without thinking it through much further, I packed up, moved back to Oregon and set up a court appearance to turn myself in. When the day came, I wore the nicest outfit I could and pleaded my case: in the time since I'd been before the court, I'd been working, taking care of my health and becoming a functional part of society. Now, I just wanted to settle all my past issues. When I was done, the judge looked quizzically at my paperwork.

"It says here this charge is from 1998, is that correct?" the judge asked.

"Yes sir," I replied. At this, he furrowed his brow in confusion.

"It's 2003," he said. "Am I to take that to mean that you absconded from justice for *five years?*" My stomach dropped a little.

"Well—yes, Judge, that's one way to put it," I stammered. "I believe technically, I've still been on probation."

"Well as of right now, your probation is completely revoked," the judge said, "and I'm sentencing you to 180 days in jail." With that, he banged his gavel and I was led out of the courtroom and into custody. *I should've just stayed in Hawaii*, I thought miserably. Instead of finding understanding and acceptance in court, I'd found the jail time I'd been trying to avoid.

I was taken to county jail to complete my sentence, though I was able to cut the time down to 120 days rather than 180 by attending a work camp. When I finished my time, I was released again, even more confused about my future than when I'd gone in. For a while, I hung around Oregon and went back to doing drugs, chasing girls and spending time with local criminals, once again feeling aimless.

After that, I moved to New York City for seven months to work for my uncle's company, where I kept doing drugs but stopped selling them. I dreamed of either becoming an actor or going back to making music. Life in New York didn't stick either, and I moved to Humboldt, California after a few months to get paid $25 an hour growing weed for a friend of mine who had been in the marijuana manufacturing business for decades.

The job paid well, and life was better than it had been in a while. I was making enough money to support myself, plus I was allowed to take home weed on credit to sell. My friend Greg invited me to stay with him in Las Vegas—and to bring marijuana, since it sold for a lot more over there. I brought my girlfriend and after just a few months, I was already developing a gambling addiction, spending all the money I was making on night clubs and party drugs.

One night, I was high on ecstasy at a nightclub in Caesars Palace, and I left my friends to hit the blackjack tables. The combination of bright lights, powerful drugs and a pocket full of money that didn't belong to me was too hard to resist. I ended up losing the $3,000 I had on me and went home to grab the rest of the cash I had stashed—though while I was there, I figured I'd take another tablet. For the next 10 hours, I was up and down like a rollercoaster, playing the high stakes tables until I finally crashed and burned.

I left the casino in the middle of the next day, my head spinning. I had started the night before with $13,000 and I had $2,500 left—none of which was actually mine, since I was in debt for the total amount. When it came time to face my friend, I lied and told him that I'd been robbed—and somehow, he believed me. Still, it was becoming clear that if I hung around much longer, something else like this would happen—not to mention the fact that I still had to pay my friend back.

Familiar thoughts were running through my head. *I need to get away from all this*, I told myself again. In 2005, I decided I was ready to skip town and head back to Hawaii—only *this* time, I would do things right.

———

Being back on Maui was a breath of fresh air, and it reminded me of the good times I'd had in the past. Once again, I started working in restaurants before meeting a customer named Jerry who put me on a different track.

"You have a way about you," he said, sizing me up. "I think you'd make a great salesman!" As he explained, I was personable and I could put my skills to better use at his car dealership. He handed me his business card and gave me some information about who to talk to and how to apply before leaving the restaurant. Sure enough, after work that day I headed to his dealership and got myself a new job.

Though there was a definite learning curve to selling cars

compared to waiting tables, Jerry turned out to be right: this was a *way* more profitable way to spend my time, and I was good at it! As my sales abilities improved, I took the job more seriously and shaped my life and schedule around it. Since working at a dealership meant keeping more regular hours and getting up early, I cut way down on my partying habits so I could keep fresh at work, limiting myself to weekend indulgences.

With my commission checks, I bought myself a nice Chrysler 300 and got a better place to live in, proud of myself that things seemed to finally be turning around. To celebrate, I went out to a club called Paradise Blues where I met a girl named Tiana. We shared a few drinks, danced and hit it off. We exchanged numbers and over the next few months, we started seeing each other regularly.

From the very beginning, the attraction between Tiana and I had been physical and in some ways superficial; she'd been drawn in by my flashy lifestyle, and we had met at a nightclub, after all. More significant, however, was the fact that Tiana's husband had died in a motorcycle accident some six months prior, and he'd left her with a four-year-old daughter named Steisha to raise on her own.

In the beginning, Tiana and I seemed to have a lot in common, and we found refuge in one another. Though she appeared to have enough money saved to take care of herself and Steisha, I gave her more security and stability, both because I made good money at my job and because I could be a role model for Steisha. For me, Tiana was a beautiful woman who could be my companion and keep me accountable. Though she drank and went to clubs when we met, she was very anti-drug, and I stopped partying so much as the two of us got closer.

Soon after we started dating I was living at her house, and in just a few months, she found out she was pregnant—which had not been in my plans whatsoever. It was a surprise to both of us, but since things were going well between us, we both wanted to keep it. I wanted to try to be a good father and a good partner, and I thought that bringing a baby into the world would help me straighten myself out even more. Unfortunately, things didn't go as planned.

While I had successfully cut down on partying to keep up with my job, one of my coworkers had introduced me to Vicodin, which I could take throughout the day to get high and still function well at work. Soon, I was secretly abusing pain pills as well. With the pressures of my relationship and fatherhood looming, I was trying to escape however I could.

I didn't have a model of what a healthy relationship should look like, and I was afraid of what I had with Tiana, not to mention our impending family. With the money I made, I avoided going home whenever I could. Instead, I would gamble and play poker, or I would go to nightclubs and get drunk. This pattern simmered for the first year or so that Tiana and I were together, but it came to a head after May 22, 2007 when our daughter Nikole was born.

After giving birth to Nikole, Tiana had to stay overnight in the hospital, and I went home to get some sleep since I'd been up all night. Seeing Coco had been one of the most beautiful experiences of my life, and I couldn't wait to get out of the hospital to celebrate becoming a father—despite the fact that Tiana was the one who had just given birth, and that I should've been there to support her.

I started by going out to a restaurant that night with my cousin and some friends to have some champagne—along with a good supply of oxycodone. Though I had no intention to stay out, I ended up going to Paradise Blues, where Tiana and I first met. I ran into a musician friend of mine who was on vacation, and upon seeing him, I flashed my hospital bracelet.

"I became a father today!" I said, slurring slightly. He smiled and congratulated me. I flashed my bracelet at everyone I met, and people bought me drinks all night long. Eventually someone brought out weed and cocaine, and after doing both, it was finally time to call it a night—in the middle of the morning. After dropping off a few buddies, I drove home to my place and blacked out.

When I came to, it was 10:30 am and someone was pounding at my door. Though I hadn't met him many times, I recognized the man as Tiana's father.

"Tiana has been trying to get a hold of you," he said, sounding concerned. Suddenly, I remembered: I was supposed to pick her up at 8 am that morning. My head was pounding and I was nauseous. With one of the worst hangovers of my life, I sped to the hospital to get Nikole and Tiana, still trying to control my nausea. Before I could go into their room, I ran directly to the bathroom and vomited for 10 minutes until Tiana came to check on me.

"Are you okay?" she asked. I was burning with shame.

"Yeah," I replied weakly. After wiping myself off, we all piled in the car and drove home. When I got home, all I wanted to do was collapse and go to sleep, but before I did, Tiana laid Coco next to me.

"Isn't she beautiful?" she asked quietly.

CHAPTER FOUR

By 2010, as Coco turned three years old, Tiana and I were fighting more and more. Things would start small and then escalate, until I could finally justify my signature move and yell, "I can't take this anymore!" before then storming out of the house.

Whenever we fought, I would eventually try to run away—and the same few thoughts would cycle through my brain. *How can she tell me what to do? I'm the provider here...I should be able to do what I want!* Of course, what I wanted to do was keep going out and partying, and stay away from home as much as I possibly could.

After months of back and forth, another fight we had made me march out of the house and get into our Lexus. Tiana followed me, scowling as I started the engine.

"Where do you think you're going?" she demanded.

"I'll be back in a little bit," I grumbled. "I just need to blow off some steam." She rolled her eyes, knowing full well that I never kept my word in these situations. Without giving her any more chances to object, I rolled up the window, backed out of the driveway and took off down the road.

I stayed up all night and into the next day partying, taking pills and drinking, topping things off with a morning golf round at Kapalua with my cousin. After golf, my cousin and I went out for dinner at his family-owned restaurant, Duke's Beach House. We hit a comedy show that night in Lahaina on Maui, which was pretty hazy through all the alcohol and the pills I'd taken. All I really knew was that the show wasn't funny, and when it was over we went out again, drinking more and flirting with all the girls we could find.

Some of my mental haze cleared at around 2:30 am, when I woke up at a friend's house, suddenly realizing that I hadn't been home in nearly two days. I decided that once the sun was up, I would start the trip back. The only problem was that to get there, I'd have to drive around the mountains, up cliffs on the Pali highway, through a tunnel, back through town and up *another* mountain to get home. In all, it would take me 40 or 45 minutes, and I was in no shape to drive.

Cramped in my Lexus on narrow, two-lane mountain highways, I was doing everything I could to stay awake and in control while fading in and out of consciousness. Partway into the drive, I called Tiana to let her know I was on my way.

"I have to get off and pay attention to the road," I slurred, the world around me getting blurry at the edges. Her voice on the other end sounded far away. It was the last image I remembered before jolting awake as my car wrapped around a light post and the airbags deployed.

My ears were ringing and the air was full of dust and smoke, debris and broken glass in every direction. I was still in the driver's seat, and the airbags had stopped me from going through the windshield. Peeking over the steering wheel, I saw the hood of the car was mangled and it looked like the engine and battery had dislodged. The car's power and computer system were dead, and the fact that I was even alive was a miracle. Then, the panic started.

The police are going to show up any second, I thought. I quickly checked the console and breathed a sigh of relief: my stash of oxycodone was still there. I shoved three in my mouth and threw the bottle into the field, scanning the scene to make out what had happened. From what I could see, no other cars were involved in the crash, and there was nobody around since it was about four in the morning. Somehow, I hadn't hurt or killed anybody. I also didn't feel injured, which seemed equally impossible.

Staggering out of the wreckage, I ran toward a nearby gas station to make a phone call before realizing I had no change. I could hear police sirens coming from about a mile up the road and I knew I didn't have much time. I spotted a cab parked at one of the pumps and walked over to the driver's side.

"Hey," I said to the cabbie, "I just got into a terrible accident, my cell phone is dead and I don't have any quarters for the payphone. Can I use your phone?" The driver looked a little alarmed, but he handed me his phone anyway. I called Tiana, and she picked up after just a couple rings.

"Where are you?" she asked, annoyed. As quickly as I could, I explained everything I could piece together about the accident before she could say anything else.

"The police are down here and I need to hide," I said finally. "I need you to come get me, *please.* I'm going to be in the bushes behind Carl's Jr." With that, I got her confirmation, gave the phone back and went to hide.

Crouched in the bushes, I could hear the sirens pass the gas station and pull up at the car wreck I'd left behind. Guilty thoughts were swirling through my head. *Tiana's ex-husband died in a motorcycle accident*, they said, *and now you're putting her through this? Right after you two just had a child together?* I felt sick.

After what seemed like forever, Tiana finally pulled up with Coco asleep in the backseat. As soon as I climbed inside and she started pulling away, I couldn't control my stomach any longer and started throwing up out the passenger's side window, passing the police cruisers as I did it. *Here I am, strung out and throwing up in front of Tiana again*, I thought, having flashbacks to the day Nikole was born.

As soon as we got home, I called the police and reported my car stolen to cover myself. When they came question me later, I lied and somehow got away with it. All through the next few days, Tiana chewed me out non-stop and I knew I deserved it. If I didn't get myself under control, I would lose my family— and maybe even my life. I was even starting to scare myself.

"I know you're mad at me," I told Tiana finally, "and I completely understand. This is getting out of control, and I know I need to make a change. I promise you, this will never happen again." Though she wasn't sure at first, I assured Tiana that I meant what I said and repeated those words like a mantra: *never again, never again.* It was a promise, and I meant it. The only problem was that my addicted mind didn't agree.

As soon as I got the call from my insurance company that they could cover the accident—even after I'd fled the scene, lied and manipulated my way out of a hit-and-run DUI—the voices started creeping back in. *You just had a bad night*, they said. *It was just because of the pills. You just can't mix Xanax with oxycodone and liquor anymore...*

I broke my promise to Tiana just three days later and went back to partying again, while Tiana's opinion of me sank lower and lower.

Even though I knew I was heading for a dead-end, even though I had two little girls at home and a girlfriend who I left alone to take care of them, I couldn't stay home. Whenever I tried, something inside me started itching until I got up and ran. I was self-destructing, and I was taking my family down with me.

CHAPTER FIVE

Shortly after the car accident and breaking my promise to Tiana, I agreed to go to treatment for the first time, and Tiana agreed to stay with me. I had become a daily OxyContin addict. Things were getting worse and worse between us, but there was still a glimmer of hope that I would get better and start being there for our family.

Though I'd seen plenty of 12-Step meetings as a kid, this was my first time actively participating in them, and so I started to see them differently. I attended Hazelden Treatment Center in Newberg, Oregon and the people there didn't seem so different from me. Even though I thought I didn't belong, I listened as much as I could and tried to grit my teeth and apply the lessons. Finally, after years of relapses, to everyone's surprise I put together 30 days of sober time. I certainly wasn't out of the doghouse, but Tiana was as encouraged by my progress as I was. *Maybe I can turn this around yet*, I thought.

Around the same time, my friend Jake was having a wedding in Los Angeles, and my other friend Todd and I made plans to attend. Since Todd was also sober, our plan was to support our mutual friend while supporting each other—but it all went out the window as soon as I was in the same room as all my old friends.

Everyone started drinking right away, and I joined in automatically before I could stop myself. Later, we were taking a limo to another nightclub when someone broke out lines of cocaine on a mirror, and with hardly a moment's hesitation, I joined in as well.

"Hey, didn't you just get back from treatment?" Todd asked me uneasily.

I sat back up and wiped my nose. "Yeah," I replied sheepishly, "but I went for pills! This is totally different." Todd raised his eyebrows and nodded skeptically, looking away. Unlike me, he hadn't caved and started drinking and doing drugs the moment we touched down in LA.

Like every other time I overindulged with friends, I soon blacked out and lost all memories of the whole weekend. I know I stayed up all night with zero sleep, drinking and doing blow with the wedding party. A girl I'd met from the bridal party gave me a ride to my hotel at around 7 am. I'd headed to the wedding with $1,500 to my name—but at the ATM, my bank balance now read zero, and the shuttle from Anaheim to LAX cost $100. Once again, I had to call the First National Bank of Grandma for help, with my flight just two hours away. Fortunately, she transferred me some cash to leave LA, tail tucked between my legs. *You were just in a treatment center that cost $27,000*, I thought as the plane took off. *And here you are two weeks later, completely destroyed.*

After getting back from LA, my relationship with Tiana got worse and worse—all the way into the beginning of 2011. Eventually, we were both unfaithful without even bothering to hide it from each other. Over the course of that year, we regularly broke up and got back together again for the sake of our family. All the same, it was clear that neither of our hearts were in our relationship, even if we couldn't let go.

I kept promising to change, and I'd get sober for a few days here and there, but overall, my drinking and drug habits were getting worse. As I felt myself losing control of my life, the idea of returning to Bend, Oregon to make a real try at sobriety became more appealing. Finally, in early 2012, I told Tiana my plans and left Hawaii to go get treatment again. Our relationship was in a worse place than it had ever been. Even so, she promised to take care of Nikole and Steisha, and that she'd support me as I tried to get help.

Back in Bend, I was more determined than ever to clean up my act, and I borrowed some money from my grandma to get back in rehab. For the first month or so, I stuck to my plan, went to 12-Step meetings and worked the steps with the sponsor I'd met, Sean G.

To pass the time and stay out of trouble, I started golfing with my Uncle John. John was my mom's youngest brother and he was only eight years older than I was, so in truth he was more like a brother than an uncle. He'd had his own struggles with addiction in the past, and he had something like five DUIs on his record. Though he wasn't out of control in those days, he'd recently been having some health issues.

On one of our outings, John wasn't hitting the ball very well, which was strange, since he was usually a much better golfer than I was. He started having trouble balancing, and then his nose started to bleed.

"You okay, John?" I asked him, helping him to sit down and catch his breath.

"I have a terrible headache," he replied. "I'm kind of dizzy." We cut our afternoon short and John rushed to the hospital to get himself checked out. Upon examining him, the doctors determined that he had glioblastoma, an aggressive form of brain cancer that was often fatal. From there, they rushed him into surgery. When it was all over, the doctors sent him home to recover with some prescription painkillers, telling us that it was an extremely aggressive cancer that was 99 percent fatal. Essentially, it was a death sentence.

As horrible as the news was, I was grateful to be in the right place at the right time. John was important to me, and he was going through the most difficult time of his life—just as I was. Still, I was dedicated to staying sober and cleaning up my act, which meant that I would have a lot of time to check up on John and take care of him. It was another reason to stay in Oregon for a while, which would only help my chances at recovery.

Before I knew it, I had a full 50 days sober and called Tiana to update her on my progress.

"I'm really doing it this time," I told her excitedly. "When I get back home, things are going to be different, I know it." After pouring my heart out, there was a pause on the other end. Something had changed.

"That's great, Nick," she replied. "I'm glad you're working on your sobriety."

"Well, I'm doing it for us," I continued, confused. "You know that, right?"

"You need to do it for yourself," she said. "I don't think there can be an 'us,' anymore. You've been gone a while, and I met someone else. The girls and I are going to move in with him." Hearing this, my ears started ringing.

"What are you talking about?" I demanded. "You can't do that!"

"I'm sorry, Nick, but it's already done," she said finally. "Just keep working on your sobriety, it's the best thing for everyone. When you're ready, I'll send the girls out for a visit."

I was so angry that I started shouting, yelling at her that I couldn't believe she was taking my kids away and that she was selfish—but when I stopped to catch my breath, I realized she had already hung up and I hadn't noticed. Even more frustrated and ashamed, I started to shake and cry.

Despite all our problems, Tiana's news had broken my heart—but why was I surprised? I had been trying to escape our family forever. We had always been "together" up to that point, no matter how shaky it was, and I always believed we would heal and come together again as a family. Now, that fantasy was gone.

Feeling furious and lower than ever as I got off the phone, I headed over to my Uncle John's house to check in with him and commiserate, stewing the entire way there. His door was unlocked when I arrived, so I let myself in and found him sleeping on the couch. No one else was around, and suddenly an idea popped into my head: *Why don't you go check out the bathroom?*

On autopilot, I walked quietly through the house to the bathroom, opened the cabinets, and there it was: yellow prescription bottles of hydrocodone. Even though I had 50 days sober, I couldn't resist. I popped the bottle top, swallowed two of his 10 mg hydrocodone pills and put everything back the way it was.

At first, it took the edge off and felt like no big deal—but then I was going back to his house every day to steal a couple more pills. Soon there weren't enough pills left for either of us, and I graduated to stealing his Lorazepam as well—until my grandmother figured out what was going on and hid his medications where I couldn't find them, keeping me from being unsupervised at John's house.

I called up old friends to find other outlets and started drinking, taking whatever drugs I could find and going to strip clubs, anything to help me forget that I was alone and living in my grandparents' spare bedroom. My addiction was taking over again, and as Johnny got sicker, so did I—but it was when I started using meth that things got much worse.

I'd used many different kinds of drugs over the years, but developing a daily meth addiction was a significant escalation. After trying it with some friends, I started using with co-workers (one of which ended up becoming my dealer). It was the most effective thing I'd found to blast the bad feelings away, ignore my responsibilities and let me focus only on the present —but it also turned darker faster than anything I'd ever experienced, and soon I needed to use it every day.

Despite everything that was going on, Tiana still had plans to send Nikole and Steisha to visit me over Christmas break, though all the while my addiction was tightening its grip. *I just need to stop using before the girls get here*, I kept thinking to myself as the weeks flew off the calendar. *I'll stop in October.* Then it was *I'll stop in November,* and finally *I'll stop in December.* Sure enough, December came, they both arrived and I hadn't stopped using. Instead, I resolved to keep it hidden as best I could, though anyone could see that something was wrong from my emaciated appearance.

The girls flew back home after two weeks of Christmas vacation, and my depression and addiction got darker. *If you can't even get sober for your daughters*, I thought, *how are you going to get sober at all?* My dreams of recovery were far in the past and I was back to taking whatever drugs I could find, every day, in full force. Soon, I was waking up early in the morning (after nights when I'd actually slept) and telling myself: *I'm not going to do this. I'm not going to do this again.* But eventually, my irritability and anxiety would become so intense that I had to put *something* in my system, just to quiet the roaring in my head.

On one of my worst benders, I used crystal meth almost

non-stop for seven days straight and went into a full panic, feeling like I might crawl out of my skin. I smoked some weed to try to calm down and my body started to seize. I couldn't talk or unclench my hands. The walls were closing in, and I could barely move. I had overdosed.

I knew I was severely dehydrated from not drinking water or eating, and my body was shutting down. I was too scared to call the paramedics because I thought I would get in trouble. Instead, I called my mom and explained the situation as best as I could, even though I could barely speak.

"I think I'm dying," I told her in a strained voice.

"You're being dramatic," she replied.

Once I pulled myself together enough to move again, I drove to her house on the freeway, hugging the right side of the road and going 25 in a 60 miles per hour zone the whole way, while snow fell lightly from the sky. Finally, I pulled up to her house and limped inside, where she settled me on the couch. She gave me a couple muscle relaxers and some anti-anxiety medication, and I lay there twitching all night, wondering out loud if I should dial 911 while she shouted at me not to call anyone.

I finally fell asleep for about six hours and woke up feeling a little better. Of course, the first thing I did when I woke up wasn't eat breakfast or drink some water. Instead, I found my mom's stash and snorted another line of crystal meth.

As I got in my car to drive away from my mom's house, I couldn't believe that I was right back where I started when I left Maui in the first place. I'd managed to put together 50 days of sobriety before dropping out of treatment, but then I'd relapsed and stopped calling Sean G. Now, I was a full-blown meth addict. Having damaged my relationships with my grandparents, my uncle and everyone else in Oregon, I started getting that familiar feeling again. *I need to start over*, I thought.

I need to go home and get clean again, but this time, I need to do it right. After seven or eight months of non-stop drug and alcohol abuse, I knew I needed another change.

I was 33 years old, unemployable, on the verge of homelessness and completely broken—financially, spiritually, emotionally and physically. I needed to make things right by Tiana and my daughters, and get my life back on the right track. In January 2013, I made the decision. It was time for me to return to Maui.

CHAPTER SIX

In the past, anytime I'd done a "geographical" (as the folks in AA meetings call it), I usually got some period of clarity and traction in a new and positive direction, even if moving to a new place didn't solve all my problems at once. This time, when I touched down in Maui, there was no rosy transition period. I had already lost too much, and I didn't have anything to start over with.

Tiana was shocked at how bad things had gotten, and it made her want to keep the girls even further away from me. Before, I'd been able to see Nikole and Steisha periodically, even if I was being kept at arm's length. Now, Tiana had full custody of them both and I was completely forbidden from seeing them unless I got sober.

Since I was too strung out to get a job, I had no money to get a place of my own—and any money I did get immediately went to drugs. I called the few friends I had left to crash on their couches when I could, but when that wasn't possible, I was sleeping on the street and stealing what I needed to survive. What I hadn't accounted for was that one of the stores where I'd been shoplifting had security cameras, and they'd been keeping tabs on me. One day, they caught me red-handed and called the police.

When I appeared in court, everything seemed all too familiar. I was exhausted.

"Mr. Terry, you're facing two felony shoplifting charges," the judge said, "and each of these counts carries a recommended sentence of five years." Just like that, the prospect of spending 10 years in prison was staring me in the face. "But after reviewing your case file, I'd like to make an alternate suggestion."

As he explained, the judge understood that I'd been going through family difficulties and had made multiple attempts in the past to get sober and improve my situation. With that in mind, he offered to extend my sentencing for a few months so that I could spend 90 days in a treatment program as my last shot at sobriety.

"After those 90 days," the judge continued, "your circumstances may have changed, and we can re-evaluate your sentencing accordingly." Hearing his words, I took a quick mental inventory of my life. I hadn't seen my daughters in six months and had completely lost the privilege of being in their lives. Every day, I was using crystal meth, drinking at least a fifth of alcohol and using opiates and Xanax when I could find them. I had no other choice. This attempt at rehab was my last chance.

After I committed to the program and got approval from the courts, I convinced my grandfather to pay for this final attempt at treatment. Everything was in place. I was scheduled to fly from Maui to Kona to attend the program when the treatment center called me.

"We know you're scheduled for 90 days, but we only have a slot in the 30-day program," one of the admissions staff explained. I was confused, but accepted the slot and flew to attend the shorter program, figuring there would be more explanations when I got there.

The rehab was called Hawaii Island Recovery, and it was on the west side of the Big Island. The property was luxurious and had a humongous pool, as well as ocean views and a chef. Right away, my spirits rose seeing how much nicer the place was than I'd expected. Still, I tried to force myself to remember what was at stake. The rehab might've looked like a place to send people who were rich and successful, but in reality, I was homeless and unemployable.

Like other programs I'd attended, every day we participated in group therapy, one-on-one counseling and meetings where we worked the 12 Steps. Early on, I was introduced to my new sponsor, Phil, who'd been recommended to me by Russell, the program manager of Hawaii Island Recovery. Phil was a recovering con artist, manipulator and street hustler who had six years clean and sober. As I soon learned, being paired with Phil was good for me, because his background helped him see through my stories. He knew how full of shit I was.

After working the program for three weeks, I was still waiting for someone to explain what would happen to me next when I found out the truth: the entire program was going out of business.

"I'm on the board of a state-funded sober living program called Bridge House," Phil explained. "It's full of people who got there through the criminal justice system, whether it's drug courts, parole or some other way. The house has beds available, so one of them is yours if you're ready to finish out your 90 days."

Though I nodded along, in my mind I saw a perfect opportunity to exit stage left. *The treatment center is going out of business!* I thought. *I can get my own little apartment, keep going to meetings, work with my mentor and do the recovery stuff on my own. I'll let the courts know the treatment center went out of business, but I don't need to be in any extended sober living program.*

Everyone in my life at the time—family members, mentors, therapists, people that I had met in AA and anyone else who knew my story—told me that going to the sober living home was my only real option. I was the one person who didn't see this clearly.

I had a list of reasons why I needed to do it my way: I was a father, I had to make money and I had to hold up my end of a relationship. Of course in reality, the only way I'd manage to do any of it was to surrender and move in an entirely new direction, even if I couldn't see it.

With about three weeks sober, I was trying to strategize how I would go against everyone's advice and get myself a condo. Throughout my life, my grandmother had always helped me come up with the first and last month's rent on new apartments, so I gave her a call and launched into my whole song and dance about how the rehab was going out of business and that I couldn't fulfill my 90-day commitment anymore, even though I wanted to.

"Well, you better go to that sober living place your sponsor suggested, then," she said. "That sounds like the best option." Internally, I groaned. *Not her, too,* I thought.

"Grandma, I would love to," I said, "but I'm not sure it's a good idea. The people up there are sketchy, and I've heard people use crystal meth there and they don't keep an eye on things. I just don't want to jeopardize my sobriety or my recovery."

At that moment, I realized how fluently I spoke the language of manipulation. I'd come up with the lie completely naturally and without rehearsing it. It wasn't premeditated; it just came out of me. I had even impressed myself!

"I'm not going to help you get a condo," she replied finally. "I don't care what you do, but the only thing I'll help you with is getting into that sober living program, or maybe another one somewhere else. But I will not finance you living on your own. Your commitment was to stay 90 days in a program, and I'm going to hold you to that." I wasn't sure if she had gone to an Al-Anon meeting or was just sick and tired of my bullshit, but for the first time, the First National Bank of Grandma was closed for business.

That night, I was still in disbelief about what my grand-mother had said on the phone. I was in an AA meeting, listening to someone share that he had struggled to be honest his whole life and had often deluded himself into believing his own lies. The man explained that he would always turn the tables on people, out of fear and to manipulate situations to get the outcome he wanted.

"By the end of it all," he said, "I had manipulated everyone and everything—and eventually, there was nothing left to manipulate." His words were like a punch in the gut.

In my many attempts at sobriety, I had heard that everyone has three voices: one in their head, one in their pants and one in their heart (or soul). For most people, the voices from the head and the pants came through loud and clear, while the voice from the heart was a whisper. On top of being loud, the voices from the head and pants tended to lie, while the whisper from the heart always told the truth. The problem was, it was almost impossible to hear the heart beneath the other voices.

Until that point in my life, everything I'd ever done had been governed by my two loudest voices. My heart would whisper things occasionally, but I would never follow its advice: either it was too quiet, or I would brush it off. But at that moment in the meeting, my heart spoke up in a clear, unmistakable tone:

You're doing it again, Nick. You're doing it again, and you can't do it anymore.

As I heard the other man share, I had an epiphany. I couldn't lie to myself or manipulate people anymore. I couldn't keep following the loud voices I'd always followed. After the meeting was over, I approached Phil.

"If there's still a bed up at that Bridge House," I said, "I'll take it."

CHAPTER SEVEN

Without a doubt, the transition from Hawaii Island Recovery to Bridge House was a shock to the system. There was no giant pool and no chef. Instead, there were dirty carpets, chores to do and cramped bedrooms that housed five people each. Even though I was homeless, unemployed and had felony charges pending against me, I was still the kind of person who could look down on people from the gutter, which was exactly what I was doing.

My alcohol and drug-induced insanity was so acute that all I could think of was the delusional idea that it might still be possible to relive my "glory days" after everything was over. I fantasized about the days when I was young in Maui and still going to nightclubs, or days when I was selling cars and still had a little money in my pocket. I hadn't had any experiences that remotely resembled a party in years, and I wanted to make a triumphant comeback. What's more, I wanted everyone who left me out in the cold to feel ashamed for kicking me while I was down (*especially Tiana*, I thought). Fortunately, whenever I started talking that way, Phil was around to remind me that the point of recovery wasn't to get back at anybody. Revenge wasn't for us.

From January 2014, Phil and I started working through the steps together in more detail than I ever had before. For about three weeks, we paid particular attention to Step Four: taking a fearless moral inventory of my life.

"The first part is to write a list of all the people you've ever resented, at any point in your life," Phil said. "Start with your earliest memories, then go through childhood, adolescence and up to the present moment." He pulled out a sheet of paper. "Then, in different columns write down what happened, who was affected and what your part in it was."

I did as Phil said, and I discovered a lot of resentments I was unaware of. Starting from the top, I wrote down my mom and my dad before continuing to my grandparents, cousins, institutions, exes and countless other people I'd encountered over the years.

In the next column, I had to list the harm I had done to others. I made a full list of the people I had harmed throughout my life, either physically, emotionally, spiritually or financially. For me, those harms included stealing, lying, manipulating and cheating—anything I could remember that had caused harm, suffering or pain to another individual. Finally, I had to list all my sexual misconduct in a fourth column.

With the first part of the exercise done, Phil and I returned to the list I'd written and talked about it repeatedly. At the top of my list was my mom, who I blamed for not being there for me; for not being the kind of mother I thought I needed; for using drugs; for having a lot of dysfunctional, codependent and toxic relationships and for not providing me any safe space as a child.

"How old was she when you were born?" Phil asked me.

"Eighteen," I replied.

"Did she ever struggle with mental health or substance abuse challenges of her own?" I replied that she had. "Did she ever get to experience the gifts of spirituality and recovery?" I shook my head no. Phil looked at me with empathy and compassion.

"Jeez," he said, "that must have been really hard for your mom—to be depressed, to suffer from alcoholism and addiction and to have never been able to experience the freedom of recovery. To me, it sounds like she did the best she could with what she had. And we need to pray for her like we would for any suffering individual."

I did as I was told, but it was hard to swallow. I loved my mom, but it was hard not to look at her from the self-centered, self-pitying perspective I was used to. I had never put myself in her shoes or tried to see things through her eyes, to understand her struggles and pain. I had always blamed her instead of trying to relate to her struggles.

My mother is an intelligent, extremely talented and beautiful soul. She is an amazing cook and because of her, I sampled all kinds of different foods as a child, things like sushi, crab, clams, mussels and all sorts of exotic seafood. She also introduced me to music from a young age, including Robert Cray, The Police, The Beatles, Sade, Prince and The Rolling Stones, all of them artists who have shaped the person I am today. When I was in the fifth grade, she worked as a radio personality doing the weather and traffic on KFOX, the only urban R&B and hip-hop radio station in Seattle. Through her job, we would get concert tickets to see artists like MC Hammer, Bell Biv Devoe, Salt N Pepa and Janet Jackson. Their live performances mesmerized me, and I immediately became a rap fanatic, which led me to becoming a hip-hop artist in my own right.

My mom supported my musical gifts and always allowed

me to be my most authentic self—but since she was my mother, I thought she owed me certain things. Now I saw that by holding onto my resentments, I was only keeping myself stuck. If I couldn't forgive her, I couldn't let it go—and if I couldn't let my resentment go, then I wouldn't be able to forgive myself for my own mistakes in life.

I hadn't realized it before, but I had been resenting myself for most of my life. I was full of shame from my own misconduct, and for how I'd treated my daughters. I blamed it all on my mother for the way I was raised, but I was re-living, re-feeling and re-enacting all the same behaviors with my kids.

When I was in my early 20s, I would stay up all night doing cocaine and other substances, reliving my childhood traumas and talking about them with my friends. At the time, I always told myself that I would never do to my own kids what my parents did to me. Now, here I was: history had repeated itself through resentment and shame.

Through the inventory process, I took each of my resentments and examined them from a new perspective. Who were the people I resented, and who had harmed them? What was their childhood like? I thought about my father and his nine brothers and sisters. He came from an abusive, alcoholic and dysfunctional family. Sexual trauma, sexual abuse and misconduct were rampant.

For the first time in my life, instead of blaming my father and shaming him for his bad behavior, I started to forgive him. I began to feel compassion and empathy for him, and I took that same approach with everybody else on my list. Slowly but surely, my resentment was transforming itself into forgiveness.

The next portion of the inventory was to write out all the harms I'd done to others. I started that list with my abandoning my daughters because of my substance abuse issues, along with lying and cheating on Tiana. Next, I wrote that I had lied, cheated and stolen from my grandparents. I had lied to my employers, manipulated my cousin and lied to him. There were so many people I had cheated and lied to, over the years.

After that list came the sexual misconduct—manipulation, things that happened when I was intoxicated and the people who were harmed. Like my list of harms, this one was long and difficult to look at.

"Did you leave anything out of the list?" Phil asked me. I said that I hadn't. "Okay," he replied. "I'm going to take a walk for about an hour. You just sit here and ponder on what we just did. When I come back, we'll finish the rest of the process."

After he left, I sat there alone next to the ocean, at the old Kailua Kona airport, feeling a lot of shame. I rehashed the memories of abandoning my daughters, stealing from my grandmother, lying to my grandfather, burglarizing my friend's home to try to steal drugs. I looked back at all the harm I had caused to the people I loved.

As I was sitting there having an inner dialogue, I started trying to talk to the spirit of the universe, or God. *What am I supposed to do with all this stuff?* I asked. *What am I supposed to do?*

In response, I heard a quiet voice rise inside me: *Let it go. Let it all go. Give it away; give it over; turn it over. Give it to God.*

With nothing else to do, I listened. I had a moment of complete surrender, releasing all my character defects and letting go of the harm I had done to others. For a moment, the weight that I had been carrying my whole life lifted—the resentment, the imprisonment of fear and the suffocation of shame—and as I looked out on the ocean, my eyes filled with tears.

About 10 minutes later, Phil came back and we continued.

"Next, I want you to write down a full list of all your fears," he said, producing another sheet of paper. Like before, I went through every fear I could think of: never getting sober, being a bad father, never having a meaningful relationship. Becoming homeless or going to prison, being alone. Fear of dying, and also of living. Fear of commitment, fear of intimacy, fear of success, fear of love. I put them all on the list. Just as the first inventory had shown me that I was living in constant shame, the second list showed me I was also living in a constant state of fear.

"This is a great list, Nick," Phil said. "I had a similar one for my fear inventory." As he went on, he said that if I continued to live my life the way that I had been, all of my fears would most likely come to fruition. "If you follow the rest of this process," he continued, "and you keep living a life of spirituality and recovery, centered in being of service to other people, I don't think any of these fears will come true." Just hearing him say that gave me a glimmer of peace.

Finally, Phil pulled out the Big Book and flipped to the Sixth and Seventh Steps. Together, we read the Seventh Step Prayer:

My Creator, I am now willing that you should have all of me, good and bad. I pray that you now remove from me every single defect of character which stands in the way of my usefulness to you and my fellows. Grant me strength, as I go out from here, to do your bidding. Amen.

When it was over, Phil smiled at me.

"Great work today, Nick," he said. "Listen, what we learned today is that you're not just an addict. You're actually a very sick person, spiritually speaking. If you're going to recover, you have to fix that, and there's a simple way to do it: you're going to need to help a *lot* of people."

Since I had so little money, I'd been driving a scooter around the island, and I'd been unable to give anyone a ride. As I saved more and more money from working odd jobs, I was able to buy a used 2010 Dodge Caravan, which I chose because it was an eight-seat passenger van. Phil had given me an assignment: to transport as many people as I could between sober living homes and 12-Step meetings—and to not charge them any gas money.

As brutal as the process was, I could feel my spirit getting lighter every day. In the past, I would never in a million years have chosen to drive around a "soccer mom van." But something inside me was shifting. As I was letting go of parts of my past, I was reconnecting with the world around me and discovering that I actually wanted to help other people. In the process, the way I acted in everyday situations was changing as well.

When I was about four months sober, I was helping a guy named Rob who I'd met through 12-Step meetings. He only had a couple of weeks sober, but he had a well-paid job; meanwhile, I was still a waiter, living on tips and essentially broke. After going to a 7 am meeting together, I suggested that we get breakfast afterwards—but as soon as we got in the car and started driving, I started feeling insecure. *You know you don't have any money to pay for breakfast*, I thought. Without thinking, I started talking.

"Hey man, I just realized something," I said. "I actually forgot my wallet at home—sorry about that. Do you mind if you pick up the tab this time and I'll pay you back later?

"For sure, no problem," Rob agreed. *That was a lie*, a voice inside me said. Now I was feeling more than just insecure: I also felt inadequate and ashamed. I kept driving, but guilt was eating me up inside the entire ride. *This guy is brand new to recovery and I have four months sober*, I thought. *I'm supposed to be more spiritually evolved than this. I shouldn't be lying to him.* Finally, when we got to the restaurant, I looked Rob right in the eyes.

"Hey, brother," I said, "my wallet isn't at home. It's right here in my pocket." I pulled it out to illustrate my point. Rob looked incredibly confused.

"I don't have any money on me right now," I continued. "I was being dishonest because I'm embarrassed about being broke, but if you pay for breakfast this morning, I will gladly return the favor the next time I get paid—that part was true."

"No problem, man" he said, with a slight chuckle. "It's not an issue—don't even worry about it." It clearly meant nothing to him, but to me, that moment meant everything. I hadn't let myself off easy like I always did. Instead, I recovered my sense of integrity and did the right thing. I'd also discovered a new tool I could use: even if I slipped up momentarily, I could always reverse myself if I accidentally told a white lie. I ended up telling on myself a lot, which was embarrassing and liberating at the same time. I learned that a half-truth was a whole lie, and that most of my life had been based on half-truths. It became abundantly clear to me: if I was going to stay sober, I needed to become rigorously honest.

CHAPTER EIGHT

By July, I had six months sober, an all-time record for me. And that's when my family called to break some sad news: my Uncle John had passed away. Since he'd died while I was in Bridge House, I'd never gotten a chance to go back to Oregon to see him, which broke my heart.

"We were wondering if you might share some words of remembrance for him at the service?" my grandmother asked me over the phone. "You two were always so close, and since you never got to see him, it might be a great way for you to say goodbye and honor the family." I was overwhelmed with gratitude that they would even ask me, and at the possibility that I might redeem myself. Without hesitation, I told them I would do it—even if it meant leaving my safe recovery bubble on the island and venturing out again into the real world.

I was worried that when I flew back to the mainland, I'd get too nervous and start drinking in the airport. In the past, I'd never done well at airports. I called my sponsor to talk about it and together we prayed for safety and protection.

When the big day came, I drove to the first airport in Kona

and was ready to fly to Oregon, but first there was a two-hour layover in Seattle—and all I could think about were the bars. Waiting in the Seattle airport, I sat on my hands and focused everything on trying not to drink, when someone walked up right behind me.

"Nick," he said. "How are you doing, man? What are you up to?" I couldn't believe it: it was my old sponsor, Sean G.!

"Sean!" I nearly shouted, giving him a hug. "What are you doing here?"

"I'm on business in Seattle and just made the last flight," he said. "It's normally a flight I never take actually, but I'm glad I did."

"It's so good to see you, man," I said. "I'm six months sober. I'm here to go to my Uncle John's funeral and to share some words on behalf of the family." Sean knew my Uncle John from meetings, and he sat down next to me as I explained everything that had happened since we last spoke.

When it was time to board the flight from Seattle to Bend, Sean and I rearranged our seats so we could sit next to each other and share stories the whole way. It was just the relief I needed to calm me down and take my mind off drinking. As unbelievable as it was, I had finally decided to let go and to pray for protection—and almost on cue, the universe had put Sean right in my path when I needed him most.

When we landed in Bend, Sean and I swapped numbers, promised to stay in touch and parted ways. Soon after, I got a message on Facebook from an ex-girlfriend of mine named Christy:

So excited to see you today!

Christy knew my uncle, and we'd gotten in touch before the trip. After seeing a post I'd written on Facebook that I was sober and coming to Bend, she'd given me a call.

"I'm sober now as well!" she said. "I'm going to be driving

from Eugene to Bend that weekend, so I'd love to get together. Maybe we can go to John's funeral together too?" I'd agreed, relieved to have another sober person I knew with me in Bend. The only problem was that when she came to pick me up from my mom's house, she showed up with a 22-ounce can of beer.

My face fell. "I thought you said you were sober."

"I am sober," she said brightly. "I haven't used heroin in eight months!"

"Oh my goodness," I replied. "Okay, well, I guess everybody's definition of sobriety is different." As we got in her car and started off together, I saw that she also had a bottle full of Klonopin in her bag—the same kind of anti-anxiety medication that I loved. They were definite red flags for me, but instead of acknowledging them or setting clear boundaries, I decided to ignore them.

We got into Bend the night before John's funeral, so I hung out with her and her friends at a local sushi bar. Later, the place converted into a dance floor with a DJ and a bunch of people crowded in to listen. It was the first time I'd been to a bar since getting sober, and since I wasn't drinking, the environment felt more and more obnoxious to me as the night wore on. To keep my energy up, I drank non-stop Red Bulls and made countless trips to the bathroom.

Finally, Christy and I ended our night at about 2:30 am and we both fell asleep. I woke up the next morning with a headache from all those Red Bulls, and from not getting a good night's sleep.

"Hey, Christy," I asked her. "My head is killing me and I'm feeling really nervous—maybe I should take one of your Klonopin before I do this speech. It might help with the anxiety and make me feel a little bit better. Even just half a pill could be helpful."

"Are you sure it's a good idea?" she asked. I took a moment

to think about it and swallowed hard, taking in a deep breath. I thought about all the times that I had tried to stay sober. I thought about everything that had transpired before, from near-death experiences, car accidents, broken relationships and all kinds of other destruction I'd caused with drugs and alcohol. Finally, I looked back at her.

"Let me make a phone call," I said. I went outside and called Phil, telling him everything that had happened and that I was considering taking a Klonopin.

"Sorry I didn't call you sooner," I said.

"I'm so glad you called me," he replied. "Nick, with everything I know about you and your life, I think it's a really good idea that you *don't* take that Klonopin." After thanking him, I got off the phone. That short conversation confirmed what I already knew: of course I shouldn't take the medication. I didn't need it. I was going to do the speech clean and sober.

When the time came to step up to the podium, I was more than a little anxious. A projector screen was showing pictures of my uncle, his daughter and their life, and in the background, Israel Kamakawiwoʻole's Hawaiian version of "Over the Rainbow" was playing. As I looked around, I saw my entire family watching me, and I was flooded with emotions. After steadying myself with a breath, I started my speech.

I spoke about what John had meant in my life and what I thought he would want me to say. I did my best to fully represent our family and to say kind things on their behalf.

Finally, I closed out the speech with the St. Francis prayer:

> *Lord, make me an instrument of your peace.*
> *where there is hatred, let me bring love.*
> *where there is offense, let me bring pardon.*
> *where there is discord, let me bring union.*
> *where there is error, let me bring truth.*
> *where there is doubt, let me bring faith.*
> *where there is despair, let me bring hope.*
> *where there is darkness, let me bring your light.*
> *where there is sadness, let me bring joy.*
>
> *O Master, let me not seek as much*
> *to be consoled as to console,*
> *to be understood as to understand,*
> *to be loved as to love,*
> *for it is in giving that one receives,*
> *it is in self-forgetting that one finds,*
> *it is in pardoning that one is pardoned,*
> *it is in dying that one is raised to eternal life.*

I wasn't religious, but the prayer seemed eerily appropriate given what had transpired on that trip—from the serendipity of meeting Sean at the airport to narrowly avoiding a relapse with Christy. Taken all together, it felt like something spiritual was actually happening in my life—even if I didn't completely understand it.

CHAPTER NINE

After my uncle's funeral, I returned to my sober community in Kona feeling more optimistic than ever before. The unlikely coincidences I'd experienced during the trip felt like guidance from beyond, and I was beginning to open to the possibility of having a spiritual life through recovery. An idea kept coming up in my meetings and my sessions with Phil: if you still hold resentment for someone, you should pray for them to help transform those feelings. Though no one in particular told me to do it, I knew I needed to start praying for Tiana. No matter how much I wanted to blame her or hold onto the past, I knew I needed to pray for her new boyfriend and for my girls. I prayed that their entire situation would be happy, healthy and full of love.

Every morning after I woke up, I said these words:

Thank you for my recovery, thank you for keeping me sober and thank you for this opportunity. I pray for Tiana, Coco and Steisha that their family will be strong and healthy, and for the absolute best situation possible.

I wasn't entirely sold on "God" or anything else, but I was

beginning to see the importance of faith. To me, developing faith was as simple as trusting what I was feeling and finding a way to express it, even if it was just to myself. I may not have known who or what I was talking to, but the act of prayer was bringing my thoughts and actions into alignment, and it was making me more interested in what I could contribute to others instead of what I could take.

My life was going better than it ever had before, but some of my old habits were still hanging on. In particular, I was spending a lot of time looking for women to sleep with—only now that I was doing it completely sober, the entire process felt a little strange. Unless I was with someone I already knew, getting into the right situations often meant being in places where people were drinking or doing drugs, which I knew wasn't ideal. On top of that, the actual hook-ups were a lot more self-conscious than they used to be, and the next morning I usually left as quickly as possible.

Meanwhile, in AA, I was constantly hearing confusing advice. "Don't get into a relationship in your first year," was a mantra that came up frequently, and I scoffed at it. To me, that advice seemed punitive and unrealistic. *The only people saying that are the people who couldn't get into a relationship in a year if they wanted to,* I thought. To get some clarity on everything, I asked for Phil's advice on sex during sobriety, and when I would be ready for my next real relationship.

"Nick," he said, "most people in the recovery community suggest one year of abstinence, or one year without a romantic relationship. With you, I think three years would be more appropriate." I couldn't believe what I was hearing; I was almost offended.

"*Three years?*" I repeated, as Phil nodded smugly. I thought he had lost his mind. I'd lost my virginity at 12 years old, and sex had been a huge part of my life ever since. It gave me a sense of connection and love with other people, and it was one of the few forms of temporary emotional relief I had left now that I was sober. I explained all that to Phil.

"That might be," he replied, "but what you were doing led to superficial connections. You chasing girls is just a distraction when you need to be focusing on your sobriety. Random sex is not the solution to your spiritual illness—and right after sobriety, your first priority should be becoming a good father."

I agreed with the second part of Phil's advice, but even if I wanted to follow his rules about sex (which I didn't), I didn't know *how* to. I was like a teenager stuck in a grown man's body. By sticking to my recovery, I showed Tiana I could be trusted again and I reunited with Nikole and Steisha, which was the greatest feeling in the world. In public, I was a good dad, a supportive father and a man in recovery giving back to his community. In my private life however, I was starting to have the same relationship with sex that I'd once had with drugs and alcohol: I would tell myself I didn't want to do it, but then I would go do it anyway.

It was a process that continued for a while, during which time I amassed a long list of superficial, short-term relationships that I tried hard not to think about too much. Overall, I was managing to stay sober and be a good dad, and maybe that was enough. Still, I could feel an inner sense of dissatisfaction and emptiness that was always threatening to take control of my life again.

Around that same time in 2016, my grandfather passed away and I traveled to Bend to go to his funeral. While I was in town, I went to a local AA meeting and saw a cute, younger girl named Tera. We had lunch together after the meeting and got to know each other. As she explained, she had three months sober; meanwhile, I had two years.

We exchanged numbers and stayed in touch, keeping

connected over social media and text until two years later, when I decided to strike things up between us again. I sent her a text:

Come visit me on Maui! I'll pay for the flight over.

It was another of my old dating tricks, and as always, it worked—she accepted the offer and we started planning her visit three months in advance. Finally, when the trip was about three weeks out, we had another text conversation:

Hey Nick, before I visit, there's something I have to tell you.

As she went on to explain, she wasn't quite as sober as she'd initially let on. As it turned out, she had recently relapsed. She still wasn't doing heroin, which had been her main drug of choice, but she'd recently been to some concerts and EDM shows with friends, gotten caught up in the moment and taken some Molly (and maybe some other drugs as well). At the end, she wrote:

But I've been completely sober now for three weeks. I just wanted to let you know.

I sighed as I finished reading her long message, feeling some nervousness creep into my stomach. It was good that she'd told me the truth, but it was still a massive red flag. Before I could think better of it, I'd already sent my reply:

Girl, it's fine. Just come anyway.

When Tera arrived, we started acting like a couple right away and even got ourselves a nice hotel room. Though we fooled around a little, she wasn't interested in having sex. She seemed disinterested in any kind of physical connection with me, and was spending a lot of time on her phone, taking pictures and scrolling.

However disappointing it was that Tera wasn't as interested in me as I had thought, I still tried to make the best of our trip by taking her around the island, buying her things and trying to show her my sense of adventure. On some level, I thought maybe it would change her opinion of me—but after three days together, she caught me off guard.

"Thanks so much for showing me around, Nick," she said with a smile. "I really appreciate it, but I'm gonna get out of your hair for the rest of the day. I think I'm going to do a little more exploring on my own out here—do some shopping, hang out with friends, you know."

Confused and trying not to act hurt, I nodded and tried to smile. "For sure, that's totally fine," I said. "Go do your own thing, I'll do mine and we'll link up later." Despite pretending not to care, the truth was that I felt an incredible sense of rejection. It was a kind of pain I hadn't felt in a long time, not since getting sober. To take my mind off things, I started swiping through Tinder—and to my surprise, she was active on there as well, having updated her profile with the recent pictures I'd taken of her around Maui!

I felt like an idiot. All the time I thought she was just distracted and playing on her phone, she was actually updating her profile and looking for other guys around me to go on dates with while we were together—even after I paid for her trip to come out. I stewed in those feelings until day turned to night, and she finally called me.

"Hey, listen," she said. "I met up with some friends and we're having a good time, so I think I'm gonna stay over here tonight and hang out."

"Oh, okay," I said weakly. "Alright, well maybe we can get together tomorrow."

"Yeah, maybe," she said distractedly. "I'll text you!" With that, she hung up, and I didn't see her again for the rest of her trip. What I did see, though, were pictures of her on the beach and at nightclubs, drinking alcohol and partying with other guys, which must've been her plan all along when she'd come to Maui.

Even though my connection with Tera wasn't different from any other short-term fling I'd had, it had usually been me leaving first and holding the ladies at arm's length. I had always thought of meeting women as a way to have fun without anyone getting hurt. Still, now that I was on the receiving end of that rejection, I was devastated.

You know not to do this, I thought angrily. *You keep getting with these girls who are new to recovery or not even sober and expecting some kind of magical result. You never find what you're looking for, and you never learn, no matter what anyone tells you.* Finally, I realized it was time to actually listen to what Phil and everyone else in AA had been telling me. Something had to change.

Even if Phil's advice had been helpful, he couldn't fully relate to what I was going through when it came to relationships. I needed someone who was more like me to talk to, someone who had a lot of sober time under his belt but who also had a lot of experience with women. Finally, at one of my meetings, I found my answer in a guy named Andre.

Andre was a long-term member of the recovery community, a licensed counselor with a Master's degree and someone with a wealth of knowledge about relationships. I'd seen him in meetings for years and we'd talked here and there, but I'd never thought to ask him for help. Shortly after the Tera debacle, I approached him and let him know what was going on.

"I've been sober for four years, so I've definitely made a lot of progress," I said. "But I'm still really struggling with relationships. It's like I'm *physically* sober but maybe I'm not *emotionally* or *spiritually* sober." Andre nodded.

"Getting sober is hard enough, so congratulations on that," he said, "but it sounds like you're starting to get in touch with your pain. And now, maybe you're ready to do the *real* work." I didn't like the sound of what he was saying, but he was right.

Even though getting sober had improved everything *external* in my life, there was something *internal* that still felt exactly the same. Even with the work I'd tried to do connecting to something spiritual and greater, there were plenty of times when I still felt so empty. I didn't want to keep living the way I was, so I was willing to do whatever it took.

After our conversation, Andre agreed to meet with me once a week. As he explained, we were going to do a deep relationship inventory on my life—just like I'd done for my resentments, shame and fears. The difference was this time, we would be listing every sexual and romantic interaction I'd had since I'd been sober, and then dissecting them to find a pattern.

In all, I wrote down the names of 12 different women and the various encounters I'd had with them over the past four years. Seeing it all written down, I was almost relieved—12 women in four years wasn't so bad! Though that might've seemed like a lot to some people, it was far fewer than I'd hooked up with during the height of my partying days.

"It might not be as frequent as it was back then," Andre told me, "but the thing you have to realize is, the behavior is still the same. You're not going out to clubs and drinking and doing drugs, but judging by the patterns in your relationships and the way you meet women, you might as well be!"

Working with Andre, we went through my "relationships" one by one—which they *were*, Andre pointed out, even if I didn't think of them that way—and we broke each one down in detail. In every single encounter we looked at, I saw the same initial pattern: I approached each of the women by saying we *weren't* going to have sex, as a way to win them over and earn a sense of safety. Then, as we got more comfortable with one another, flirted more and they felt more connected to me, we *would* end up having sex—even though I wasn't spiritually or emotionally connected to them. Of course, it wasn't until Tera that I'd given any thought to how that dynamic must have felt to the women I'd been with.

I never considered the pain and damage I might have caused, that some of the women might have had sexual trauma in their lives that they were processing in a compulsive way, or that some of them might have had children. I didn't think about any of it. When I was done with a relationship, I just pulled the plug. I didn't call or text. The connection and the chase were over, so I was out.

"Nick," Andre said, "you're not okay with what this girl Tera did to you, but you did the exact same thing to these 12 women over the last four years." I sank down in my chair as he said it, but I knew he was right. In truth, none of my romantic encounters had ever felt truly *good*. All of them left me feeling empty, shallow and disconnected. At the root of it was something I had never before considered: my dishonesty and callous nature around sex.

As far back as early childhood, I had been a compulsive liar. I told other kids that my dad was famous. Throughout my adolescence and teens, I was constantly making up grandiose stories about myself and my family to hide the truth, and as an adult, I would lie and manipulate anyone and everything to avoid accountability and get my way. My sexual and romantic relationships were no different.

All of my lying, cheating, manipulating and abandonment came from a deep lack of integrity, honesty and thoughtfulness about the impact my conduct had on others. After seeing it laid out before me, I was floored.

"The question is, Nick," Andre asked, "now that you know this about yourself, what are you going to do? Are you going to keep doing the same stuff you've been doing? Or are you going to make some changes?"

"I'm going to change," I said finally. "I have to."

At nine months sober, I was proud of all the progress I'd made in recovery, but I was starting to crave more purpose in my life. Even though I wasn't being triggered or compelled to drink alcohol in my career as a waiter, I definitely wasn't loving the work. I shared this with my sponsor Phil, and like most people in the recovery community, he gave me a familiar adage: "Have you prayed about it?"

The question always made me want to roll my eyes, but since I was starting on a new path, I was more open than usual to taking direction other than my own. So, like Phil told me to, I prayed.

A few days later, I found out that the recently-closed Hawaii Island Recovery had reorganized and reopened at a new location. Some of the staff had heard I was living in the community of Kona and that I'd been staying sober and regularly attending meetings. As such, they offered me a job as an overnight tech at the center five days a week—and it felt like a dream come true.

Embarking on a career in mental health and substance abuse treatment felt absolutely wonderful to me, and as an alum of the program, I thought that I could add value to the program by sharing my experience, strength and hope with any new admissions who came in.

In my role as an overnight tech, I would arrive at 10pm, make sure everyone was settled into bed and act as a safety person for any potential overnight emergencies. Usually, what it really meant was practicing my meditation on the couch in the TV room (which in turn really meant resting my eyes).

As I progressed, I was given the opportunity to take on some part-time work with admissions as well. As part of that work, I was answering phone calls, explaining the program to families and then connecting any interested calls I got to my supervisor, Jimmy.

I loved communicating with people and sharing my story about the recovery community in Kona. All of it strengthened my passion and sense of purpose. I was finally doing work that I really had a zest for.

At about 18 months sober, I was in awe at how amazingly well my life seemed to be going. I was staying sober, finding community, developing a sense of purpose and still regularly attending support groups. Even so, there was still one thing missing. In my heart, I knew I needed to reconnect with my daughters back on Maui. Again, I shared with Phil that my heart yearned to be back in my daughter's life—and again, he had told me to pray about it, which I did.

Shortly after my conversation with Phil, I was at work in admissions fielding another call from a gentleman who had questions about our treatment program, though I wasn't sure if he was looking to become a patient or was just gathering information. After a few conversations, it turned out that I actually knew the guy from 12-Step meetings back in Lahaina, Maui—through the recovery community, he was even a friend of my dad's!

His name was Dr. Jay Searle, and after talking for a while, our conversation turned more personal. "I'm actually opening a recovery treatment program on Maui," he said. Immediately, I perked up. "You should think about coming to work for us—we could definitely use you!" As he explained, the program would be called Maui Recovery (a name that immediately resonated with multiple meanings for me). Once again, I had prayed; and once again, in typical universal fashion, my prayers were being answered.

After an interview process, I was offered the role of property manager at Maui Recovery, a beautiful, pristine property in Kihei. To get ready for my new responsibilities, I moved back to Maui on September 15th, 2015, six months before the facility was scheduled to open for business.

Though Maui Recovery hadn't opened yet, my job meant that I was allowed to live onsite and could move in early. It gave me a gorgeous place to stay—and a place to invite my daughters Coco and Steisha to come visit, where they could swim in the pool and explore the beautiful property with me.

After just a few visits, my daughters and I were starting to reconnect, and my heart felt fuller than ever. Since I was back on Maui, and Tiana saw that my life and sobriety were going well she agreed to allow me to split custody of Coco. The new parenting arrangement was that I could have Coco on Friday, Saturday and Sunday, and that I would drop her off at school on Monday, and just knowing that I'd be spending more time with my daughters made my soul smile. After everything that had happened between us, I knew mending our relationships wouldn't be easy—but I knew I was in the right place, and I was determined to do whatever it took.

***

In 2016, when I was two-and-a-half years sober, I got the news that my grandpa Jim had died. He was the most honest principled disciplined person I had ever met. He was the father figure I had in my life, and I had always honored our bond so deeply. Now that he was gone, I couldn't help but reflect on how my addiction had damaged our relationship in so many ways, and it filled me with a tremendous sadness.

Even so, I held onto the last memories I'd experienced with my grandpa Jim. For whatever had happened between us in the past, he had been so happy and proud of all the changes I'd made in my life. After his funeral, Tiana asked me if I could talk.

"I'm going through some stuff right now," she said quietly, clearly dealing with a pain that she couldn't share all the details of. "And things are so different now for you, so I was wondering...could you take care of Coco full-time for a while so I can figure some things out?"

I felt for Tiana, but I also couldn't believe what I was hearing. Since I'd gone to Kona to get sober, I'd been absent and unavailable for the first several years of Coco's life—and before that, I'd done plenty of things to damage Tiana's trust in me. But now, in a moment of need, she was trusting me again to take care of our daughter!

Even if I couldn't figure out how it all had happened, I was beyond excited for the opportunity to step up to the plate, make things right and reciprocate the love that Tiana had shown our family while I had been healing.

As I knew it would, reconnecting with Coco meant working through fear and insecurities, healing a lot of pain and putting my recovery to the test. For every hard moment we had together, I was realizing more and more that being in Kona for almost two years had changed me.

I was not the same man I was before in the depths of my addiction. Where I used to run from pain and responsibility, I was now able to receive and embrace them. I could sit in discomfort, accept responsibility and listen now. Through the 12 Steps, I was becoming more and more accountable for my actions.

Without necessarily intending to, I had started learning how to live. I was transforming into a better person—into someone who could actually be a father.

As I continued working my steps in recovery I figured it was time that I did a formal 9th step with Tiana so I reached out to her. I had asked her to make a face-to-face amends and she had declined. "The only thing I want from you is for you to do be a good father to Coco," she'd said at the time. This hurt me deeply but I knew I had to honor her request, this wasn't about me anymore, it was about making things right and cleaning up my side of the street.

What I hadn't known when I started taking care of Coco full-time was that it wouldn't be a part-time thing. After Coco moved in with me, she never moved out—and that has been one of the greatest blessings of my life.

Watching my daughter play sports, performing in plays or just dropping her at school, I sometimes still feel a pride rise up through my belly that almost feels unfamiliar. *I'm doing it,* I think in those moments, with the warm image of Steisha always rising up in my mind as well. *I'm doing the best I can to be a good father.*

CHAPTER TEN

After working with Andre, I made a firm decision to change my ways, even if it was going to be one of the hardest things I'd ever done. From that day forward, I decided I was going to set a simple new rule for myself: I would not have sex with another woman until I felt a spiritual, emotional and a physical connection with her—and *in that order*.

As soon as I decided to change my behavior, it became impossible not to see my own manipulative patterns whenever I felt the impulse to act on them. I noticed how I was looking at women on Facebook and Instagram to distract myself from difficult emotions, or to put off work I had to do. When I sent that first message, I knew I'd be able to get some kind of dopamine hit from what followed...though I also knew what kind of emotional disasters I was heading for.

Through a lot of practice, I found that if I just didn't send that first message, and if I didn't instinctively approach every woman I met who caught my eye, I didn't end up in those situations. Time and again, I kept catching myself wanting to return to my old ways, but on each occasion, I resisted. My patience increased, and I more started focusing on my own discipline. I doubled down on service and helping others, and I spent a lot more time working on my health and going to the gym.

The process of resetting all my bad habits took about a year —and then one day in May, 2019 I was at my CrossFit gym when a beautiful girl walked in. She was Asian, with dark skin, long, black hair and a toned, athletic body. She seemed like she was about five foot four, and I noticed a tattoo on her back. Since she caught me looking at her, I gave her a smile and she smiled back. After she walked away, I turned to my workout buddy and raised my eyebrows.

"If I had a girlfriend who looked like that," I told him, "I wouldn't let her leave the house." He laughed.

"She's gotta have a boyfriend or something," he said.

A few minutes later, the instructor came out and started leading everyone through that day's workout, starting with some sprints. Right in the middle of them, I noticed the same girl coming up behind me. *Oh my God*, I thought, *this crazy hot girl is right on my bumper. I can't let her pass me—no way.*

I pushed myself harder than ever to make sure she couldn't lap me, and after the sprint was over, I stopped for a minute of rest before going again. Looking around, I saw my dream girl finishing her sprint just a little behind me, and our eyes met. She knew what I was doing, and she was *definitely* trying to pass me. Just by her gaze, I could tell she had an intense, competitive spirit—and I knew that I couldn't let her win.

After seven more rounds of all-out sprints and a brutal exercise CrossFitters refer to as "toe-to-bars", she was still right on my heels, though she never got past me. I was starting to get a fluttery feeling in my stomach, which shocked me—I hadn't felt anything like that since middle school! Though we hadn't even exchanged words yet, I could sense there was an attraction building between us. I could feel it.

When the workout was over, I looked around for the girl to introduce myself but couldn't find her anywhere; she seemed to have disappeared. I went home disappointed and started investigating on Instagram, starting with the gym's social media handle. Eventually, I found her: her name was Paulina. Though she didn't have many pictures up, it was definitely the same person—and one of the few pictures on her grid was a selfie with an older guy in a suit, some Dr. Somebody who had his arm around her.

I looked closer and saw the post was only about four or five months old. My stomach fell. *Well, there you go*, I thought. *Too good to be true.*

A few weeks later, I went to CrossFit again on Memorial Day for a workout. I'd been feeling stressed, and I knew the gym was what I needed. They had "hero workouts" on holidays, which were training sessions designed to be even more grueling than usual—but after they were over, everyone hung out, celebrated and had a barbecue. It was the best of both worlds: the intense exercise would take my mind off things, and at the end there would be free food.

When I showed up that morning for my workout, my heart jumped. There was Paulina, sitting on the lawn some distance away from me. When we all finished our workout, she came up right behind me again and lay down by a fan to cool off, still panting. Seeing her so close, I walked over to her on autopilot and reached out my hand. She took it, and I lifted her up.

"Thanks," she said with a smile. *Why did you do that?* I thought. It was completely out of character, and something I normally would've only done with someone I knew really well. Shaking my head, I walked to the bathroom to get some fresh air and collect myself. When I returned, everyone was hanging out and taking pictures together to capture memories from the day. Paulina and I were in a couple of group shots, and I finally had a chance to introduce myself and make some casual conversation. Through our chit chat, I couldn't stop thinking about the picture on her Instagram. *Where's that guy you were with?* I wondered. Every time I'd seen her in person, she'd been alone.

"Are you going to the barbecue after this?" I asked her.

"I am!" she said. "I just have to run home first."

"Great," I replied. "Me too. Well, I guess I'll see you there!" She nodded and stuck her hand out.

"Cool," she said as I shook her hand. "I'm Paulina, by the way."

After running home to grab two beach chairs and my one-year-old French bulldog, Snoopy, I headed back to the barbecue and sat down in a circle with some casual gym friends. A few minutes later, I noticed that Paulina was sitting off to the side in the sand.

"You can use one of my beach chairs!" I called over to her, gesturing to my extra seat. She smiled and made her way over.

"Awesome," she said. "Thanks, Nick." As the day went on and the surf started to swell, I got up to do some body surfing. Paulina was in the middle of a conversation nearby when I approached her with Snoopy.

"Do you mind watching my dog while I go jump in the ocean?" I asked. Her eyes lit up.

"He's the cutest dog ever!" she said. "I'd love to watch him." With that, I thanked her, handed her the leash and jumped into the ocean. After I came back to get Snoopy, I took a seat near Paulina, who seemed a lot more comfortable now than she had been before. Unable to stop myself, I eavesdropped on her conversation.

She was speaking candidly to the girls around her about her recent struggles with Adderall addiction. It had helped her get things done, she explained, but she ultimately quit because it was stopping her from connecting with people, and because it made her less involved in the fitness world.

"I'm really grateful I started CrossFit and I met you guys, though," she said finally. "I just bought a home nearby and I'm in the middle of remodeling it, so I'll be over here all the time! It'll be nice to have some people to spend time with as I get back into the single life." Hearing her say those magic words, my heart started beating faster—I still had a chance after all!

A little later, I stood up and started saying my goodbyes when Paulina spotted me.

"Hey," she said, "don't forget your chair!"

"Go ahead and keep it," I replied with a smile. "I'll get it from you later."

I left the barbecue with a warm feeling in my chest, and I couldn't stop thinking about Paulina. Somehow, I knew she was the person I wanted to be with. When I got home, I followed her on Instagram—and at the exact same moment, she sent me a friend request on Facebook. I was so excited that I messaged her right away:

I just followed you on Instagram at the same time you sent me a message!

After a moment, she replied:

Well, I guess it was meant to be!

I couldn't believe my luck.

Since you're new to the island, it would be fun to take you on an adventure sometime if you're up for it?

After a moment, she replied:

I would love that!

Basking in the light of her response, I watched the text cursor blink for a moment or two. Finally, I started typing again:

I actually have a pool and a hot tub over at my place. Want to come have a hot tub tonight?

After what felt like longest wait of my life, Paulina finally replied:

That sounds good :)

We set a time for her to come over and I sent her my address. As I got my place ready, the same few thoughts kept looping through my head. *Don't blow this, Nick—don't try anything stupid. Don't try to touch her, don't even try to get inside her personal space. Just be a gentleman.*

When Paulina arrived, I kept repeating the words over and over—even louder as we got close in the swimming pool, and closer still in the hot tub. Though nothing physical happened between us, she was giving me a clear message that she was interested. Even so, I was determined that this time was going to be different. This time, I was going to do things right.

Soon after our first "date," Paulina and I started spending more time together and going on adventures. We met up at CrossFit, went on hikes together and had barbecues at my house. Things had been going well between us, but the turning point was when Maui Fest came to town, a two-day recovery convention at a hotel called the Royal Lāhainā. I had already made hotel reservations, as it fell on my birthday weekend at the end of May. The only issue was that I'd invited another girl.

I'd met Jackie right before I saw Paulina for the first time. We'd flirted a little on social media, and we had some friends in common from the local recovery community in Hawaii. Though I'd been pretty good about staying abstinent, the way I'd messaged Jackie was a lot more in line with my old patterns. Now I was panicked that my friendship with Jackie might ruin this new and intense connection I had with Paulina.

Though I hadn't known Paulina for very long, my feelings for her were strong and undeniable. I had a friendly flirtation with Jackie, but I really wanted to be with Paulina—and time was ticking to resolve the situation. *Should I invite Paulina to come with me to the convention and tell Jackie the truth,* I thought, *or should I stick to my plans with Jackie and not tell Paulina about it?*

As I weighed the two options, I could feel myself leaning towards the more dishonest choice. Paulina and I had only been talking for 10 days or so, and we hadn't made any kind of commitment to each other—I wouldn't be doing anything wrong by following through on the plans I'd already made, right?

When the day of the convention came, I checked myself into the hotel the same night Jackie was supposed to fly in. I still hadn't told either Jackie or Paulina what was going on, and time was almost up. Not knowing what else to do, I called Andre to ask for his advice and prayed on it. Finally, I decided that I would call Jackie and tell her the truth.

"Listen," I said, "I'm so sorry to be doing this, but I don't feel comfortable having you come over tonight. I just started this new connection with someone else, and I don't know where it's going, but I'm very attracted to this girl. I think it would be irresponsible for me to have you over and not tell her."

Even though Paulina and I hadn't done anything physical together and we had no history, spending a night with Jackie still felt like it was going against my values. For once, I just wanted to do the *right* thing. After I told her the truth, I braced for her to chew me out for wasting her time—but instead, she thanked me.

"It's really nice to have a man be honest and truthful for a change," she said. "Thanks for that, and don't worry about it— it's not a big deal." After hanging up the phone, I felt a huge weight lifted off me. It was the first time I had ever done something like that. Instead of trying to juggle two relationships and sacrifice my character, I just made a clear and honest choice—

and the next call I made was to invite Paulina to go to Maui Fest with me.

"I'm at this kind of spiritual convention," I said. "Basically, it's a bunch of yoga and stuff. I'm also going to have dinner here with my dad and my daughters, and it would be so cool if you could come." I was nervous—I hadn't told her I ran in any holistic recovery circles, and she definitely hadn't met my family yet, which was a big step. But she didn't even flinch.

"That sounds great!" she said. When the time came for dinner with Paulina and my family, I explained a little more about the convention and my journey to sobriety. She nodded along, listening intently.

"I actually had kind of a troubled childhood," Paulina said, "so my parents sent me to this therapeutic boarding school for a couple of years. They did all kinds of group therapy and a lot of processing. I have a bachelor's degree in psychology, so this kind of stuff fascinates me." *Oh, gosh*, I thought. *Could this be any more perfect?*

For about an hour over dinner, Paulina shared her story before we all went to a big conference hall to hear a speaker. There were a couple hundred people there in the crowd, and Paulina grabbed my hand so she wouldn't lose me. She held it through the entire talk. When it was over, we went outside, took our sandals off and walked on the beach under the stars. We sat down and I put my arm around her, trying to kiss her as she kept playfully turning the other way. Finally, when we got back to the hotel, we had our first kiss together on the beach. That night, my daughters shared a bed together and though nothing happened between us, Paulina stayed over as well.

CHAPTER ELEVEN

After Maui Fest, Paulina and I got closer, developing an even deeper spiritual connection. Since she was raised Buddhist, she taught me more about meditation, and we started practicing together. She started coming to 12-Step meetings with me, and we shared more and more aspects of our lives with one another. Through it all, our dynamic felt like a dance.

After some time, Paulina told me that she'd done a three-month retreat in France when she was 18 at Thich Nhat Hahn's monastery, Plum Village, and that it had been one of the most memorable experiences of her life. Soon after, I got an invitation from a friend of mine who worked at the Quepasana Foundation in Makena to go on a 10-day silent meditation course. The course was a gift and didn't cost any money, though the foundation encouraged donations.

It was kind of a twist on a Vipassana retreat, though it would also feature all-organic food prepared by a chef, six hours a day of sitting meditation and four hours a day of yoga. The first six days would be just for adults, but on the sixth day, kids could come and join in as well. I knew Paulina was passionate about meditation, and I also knew I wasn't very good at it yet and could use the support. So I invited her to come along, even though we'd only been dating for about two months. Her eyes lit up.

"Of course I'll come with you," she said, beaming. "Absolutely!" I hadn't thought through the implications of a 10-day silent retreat for two people who were just newly dating, but I didn't think I needed to. Though it had only been a few months, I already felt like I'd known Paulina my whole life. And after Paulina agreed to come, I enlisted my daughter Coco as well.

I hadn't read the fine print before showing up, but as the more detail-oriented person between the two of us, Paulina had read all the preparation materials.

"It says here that we're not even supposed to look at each other," she said. "They don't want us to even have eye contact." I glanced at her sideways, a little confused.

"That can't be right," I said, dismissing it—but sure enough, that was *exactly* what the organizers wanted: complete, noble silence. They wanted to create a space where people could be completely alone, while still in the presence of others. It was a tall order for two people who were starting to fall in love.

Paulina and I got settled in separate canvas tents with Airstream mattresses, and for the first two days of the retreat, I did a pretty good job. Even if Paulina and I briefly looked at each other here and there, we were mostly honoring the rules. Still, what I'd learned over the years from people who had done meditation courses was that if somebody was going to leave, it usually happened on the third day. If you could make it past the third day of a 10-day retreat, you could usually stay for the whole thing—but there was something about the third day that could break you.

Boy was that true. On the third day, my mind was spinning

and I couldn't stop thinking about Paulina. I wanted to know how she was feeling, what she was thinking about, and I wanted to talk to her. I wanted the rush of feeling connected to her again—but then I noticed that Paulina had stopped trying to return my eye contact. Now, she was focused on her meditation.

All at once, I started having a flood of doubts about coming to the meditation retreat. At the center of the property stood a gigantic tent, where an older teacher named Jorge presided over the course. He was a short, bald guy in his 60s, but he also owned the entire multimillion dollar parcel of land where we were staying, and he had an intense, magnetic aura.

The students in the front row of the tent had been part of Jorge's meditation community for a long time, and they took on a kind of leadership role. There were also a handful of younger, attractive women amongst them, giving Jorge the appearance of a guru. In the second row sat the slightly less experienced students, then in the back were all the newbies, which is where Paulina and I were sitting.

All of a sudden, my mind was racing. *Paulina had a realization while she was meditating and now she doesn't want to be with me anymore,* I thought. *Jorge and the women in the front row are going to come and ask her to join them. They're going to bring her into their meditation cult and she's going to leave me.* I was spinning all kinds of jealous scenarios out of thin air, all because Paulina was focusing on her own inner work.

Throughout the entire meditation, I kept looking over to check that Paulina was still there, and that she hadn't run off with some other student. I was losing my shit. Meanwhile, Jorge was giving us gentle instructions to disconnect our minds from our bodies.

"Be in the audience," he said. "Just observe." Hearing his voice made me remember something. Since we were only allowed to read the books that were kept at the retreat, I'd picked up *The Power of Now* by Eckhart Tolle on the first night and read some of it to take my mind off things. Tolle had also written that our job is to be the quiet observer, a witness to our own thoughts. As he explained, we will all die one day, and we will be emptied of all our attachments. None of the illusions and thoughtforms we are obsessed with in life will remain; all that will be left is silence and stillness, with our truest selves witnessing it.

All these thoughts are just my ego and attachments talking, I reminded myself. *It's not me. I have to become the observer.*

After struggling through the rest of the day as best I could, I finally went back to my tent to go to bed. That night, I had the first lucid dream of my life. While I was asleep, I told myself I was dreaming and I could wake up any time I chose to. I was in complete control. My vision became incredibly sharp and I was fully aware of my surroundings. I was fascinated by being in full communication with myself, something I had never felt before.

When I woke up on the morning of the fourth day, I felt calm and relieved. Whatever had happened in my dream the night before still lingered, and I could feel myself separated from my thinking. For the first time in my life, I had become the witness.

Just like the previous day, everyone gathered to for group meditation, and I did the same with a smile. The dysfunctional, jealous thoughts of the day before still came—but this time, I saw them for what they were. *Nick, you're doing it again,* I thought. *My God, you really think Paulina is going to run off with a 65-year-old meditation guru?* I couldn't keep a huge smile from forming on my face; in fact, I could barely hold myself back from laughing out loud. I was laughing at myself, and it was the most liberating experience of my life.

Just like the instructors had said, my thoughts weren't *my* thoughts. They were the residue from a lifetime of conditioning, insecurity, jealousy and an absence of self-love. They were the result of a dysfunctional mind, and I could separate from them. Once I did that, they lost all their influence over me. And that was powerful.

From there, I dropped into a smooth, hour-long meditation without opening my eyes for the first time. I did a full body scan and moved outside of my body before bringing my consciousness and awareness back inside. All the time, the only thing keeping me tethered to the world around me was the gentle rhythm of my breath. There was a connection between me, my thoughts, my breath and the world around me that I had never noticed before.

Between our meditation and yoga sessions, the instructors led us through some breathing exercises that were entirely new to me.

"All you need to know," one of the instructors said, "is that these breathing techniques are a way of 'getting high on your own supply,' so to speak."

The technique involved a strong inhale through the nose and an equally strong exhale through the mouth, repeated 30 or 40 times. On the final exhale, we emptied our lungs of all oxygen and stayed that way, holding our breath for one full minute. The process felt awkward and triggered strong feelings of anxiety. It almost felt like I was suffocating, but the instructors reminded us that we were okay and helped us through it.

To my surprise, they were right: I was able to hold my breath for the entire minute. In the second round, the time increased to 90 seconds, and again I made it through, despite my body telling me otherwise. In the last round, we all held our breath for *two full minutes*, the longest I ever had. Coming out of the exercise, I felt completely alive, alert and focused. It was true, I did feel a slight buzz from the oxygen rushing through my system—but this was different from drugs and alcohol. I didn't feel like I was escaping from who I was. Instead, the breathing had me sink down *deeper* into myself, past all the distractions and anxieties and down to a core sense of joy I'd forgotten about. I was consciously connected and firing on all cylinders.

"The beautiful thing is that when you leave here," one of the instructors said, "this is a practice you can and should keep doing. There's no harm in it, and it can become a regular part of your life." Hearing those words, a calmness washed over me. *This is what I've been looking for*, I thought. *This is the missing piece.*

On the sixth day, Nikole showed up and the rules of the retreat loosened. The instructors didn't want the kids to have to engage in extended silence, so they had lots of activities planned. Since the children were all playing and making noise, the adults were now permitted to start speaking quietly to one another, and making eye contact was allowed while engaging with the kids.

Paulina and I got away from the noble silence we were all consciously cultivating together by spending some time with Nikole and the other children. The instructors helped Nikole do some short meditations and play with some sound bowls. We made leis, did laughing yoga exercises and swam in the ocean. In those moments, I had never felt closer to Paulina, Nikole or myself. We were truly a family.

Finally, the 10-day course was completely over, and Paulina and I were free to talk to one another again. The process of adjusting to normal noise and conversation after so much silence was a little jarring, but it was beautiful to hear Paulina's voice again. On the drive home, I had to ask Paulina a question that had been on my mind the entire retreat.

"Remember how we were sneaking eye contact with each other for the first couple of days?" I asked her. "What was up on the third day? Why did you stop?" Her eyes widened and she smiled.

"Oh my God," she said, "you won't believe it." She told me that one of the instructors had secretly approached and confronted her about the rules of the retreat. According to Paulina, the instructor had asked her to honor the space by not making so much eye contact with me.

"She said she knew we were in a relationship, but it was distracting the other students," Paulina continued. "I felt kinda guilty, so I tried to follow her instructions. Sorry if that was weird." In response, I burst out laughing, to Paulina's great confusion.

"What?" she said with a smile. "What's so funny?"

"Nothing," I replied, after finally collecting myself. "I'm just the luckiest man in the world."

CHAPTER TWELVE

In 2020, Paulina and I had been together for a little over a year when she got a phone call that her 11-year-old cousin, Elayna, had attempted suicide. Our usual morning routine was to go down to the beach and meditate, and sometimes I'd go surfing, but that phone call stopped us. Paulina was devastated, and I didn't know how to respond. We were in the middle of a global pandemic and people weren't traveling. As an "essential worker" at the treatment center, I still had to go in to work that day. Paulina requested that we surf and meditate as usual—that was how she wanted to process the morning.

I followed her lead and we went down to the beach. I went out to surf while she kept meditating. I didn't know what to do, and I felt inconsiderate as I thought about the circumstances. When I came back in to be close to her, Paulina told me what she'd decided during her meditation. She would fly to California that night to be with her little cousin. Paulina and her cousin have a very special and important relationship. She loves her like her own daughter.

That afternoon when I got home from work, Paulina told

me she'd booked her flight for Los Angeles. Elayna was in the hospital, and she planned to stay with her until she got better. I dropped her off at the airport that night, and she was gone. As I write this, she has still been gone for five months, and our relationship has been put to the test as never before. Even so, something beautiful has happened that probably never would have transpired otherwise.

Every night during her treatment, the doctors transitioned Elayna into a pediatric psychiatric hospital where they took great care of her, and they also allowed Paulina to stay overnight. During the long weeks she was gone, that old voice of mine would sometimes come back, fading in and out like a weak radio signal. All the uncertainty was bringing back my childhood feelings of being unworthy of love, of being separate, different and alone again. Whenever those voices spoke to me, I would practice being the quiet observer and disconnecting from them, not allowing them to dictate what would happen in our relationship. I wanted to be one hundred percent supportive of Paulina's journey and put all my needs and desires to the side.

Finally, the professionals at the hospital started looking into Elayna's case. Between stay-at-home orders, family issues, doing school remotely and spending too much time on Snapchat and social media, everything had taken a physical toll. On top of everything else, her mother was struggling with substance abuse and trauma from years of experiencing domestic violence, all of which created a toxic environment that had culminated in Elayna's suicide attempt. It was no ploy for attention, and it was not attention-seeking behavior. It was clearly a real attempt to leave the planet.

Paulina had been there every day for the weeks of their family crisis, and without hesitation, she decided to sign us up to take care of Elayna and Lucy for a while so her mother could take some time to regroup. When Paulina called to tell me, my fearful, anxious thoughts came back in full force. *How long will this last? Three months, six months, 18 months? What will it all mean for our relationship?* But I put all that to the side and told Paulina that I supported her completely. Doing so was one of the best decisions I could have made.

Watching Paulina leave her life behind to take care of Elayna is one of the most attractive things I've ever witnessed. Paulina was a real estate agent on Maui juggling multiple projects, including a remodel and the construction of a new addition. She has family here, a CrossFit community and many friendships. Still, she left it all with no hesitation to be of maximum service to a beautiful 11-year-old child. Through the challenges of our five-month, long-distance relationship, Paulina stayed in a mental hospital every night and didn't even blink at committing to being a foster parent to two children, one of whom isn't related to her. It was at that moment that I decided: *I'm going to ask Paulina to marry me.*

I worked with Paulina's best friend Aundi to figure out what kind of ring she wanted, and we finally picked out a perfect diamond. Still, what I didn't expect was that all the secret plans to surprise her would also involve telling little lies here and there, which made me deeply uncomfortable. It reminded me of a life I never wanted to go back to.

When the time came, I flew overnight from Maui to Vegas, arriving at 9 am in the desert. Paulina had a medical procedure that day which would last for five hours, and I used that time to go to the jeweler and pick from three oval diamonds. The universe winked at me again that day, as Ed the jeweler announced he was 30 years sober since graduating from the Betty Ford Clinic. After a few hours, I made my choice and Ed gave me a gift certificate for a bouquet of flowers from the shop next door to give to Paulina after her surgery.

Paulina was still woozy from the anesthetic when I picked her up at the clinic, and the nurse wheeled her to the car where I helped into the passenger seat. She was shivering, so I gave her my jacket and turned the heat up. I could tell she was uncomfortable and in pain. Still, the first thing she did after collecting herself was look over at me and ask, "What have you been doing for the last five hours?"

I was caught completely off guard. I hadn't even thought of a lie or a story about where I'd been and what I'd been doing! In that moment, I realized I hadn't had to lie or manipulate in so long that I'd almost forgotten how to do it!

"I played some poker," I replied, trying to be aloof.

"Poker?" she asked, concerned.

"Yeah, honey," I replied nervously, "I played a little poker."

"Well, I hope you still have some money left," she said. *Why did you say you played poker?* I asked myself. *There's a million other things you could have said but you chose poker? What is wrong with you?* Still, after a lie comes out, you have to commit to it—so that's what I did.

Paulina and I stayed at the Red Rock Resort while she recovered from her surgery, and I waited on her hand and foot. While Paulina went out to get her nails done, I embarked on another covert operation to pick up the engagement ring. Once again, when I met up with Paulina, I hadn't prepared a reasonable story about where I'd been for an hour and a half. I was 10 minutes late picking her up, and her first question was, "Where'd you go?"

"I was meditating," I lied.

"Meditating?" she asked. "Meditating where?" I responded impulsively that I had found a nice park a few miles away, where I sat on a bench and listened to a guided meditation. She accepted my story, and again I asked myself why I couldn't make up better excuses. *You're not very good at this anymore,* I grumbled to myself.

Finally, with the perfect ring ready to present to my fiancé, I took Paulina to Mount Zion National Park for an incredible hike called Angels Landing. It was December 7th, Paulina's birthday, and we parked the car and started out on the trail. A passing hiker informed us our timing was impeccable: they had just opened the trails to the public after being shut down since March. We'd also been blessed with a perfectly crisp, sunny morning—though as it turned out, the hike I'd chosen was pretty dangerous. The sign out front explained that 15 people had died on it since 2004, and that travelers should use caution since there were no shuttle buses to transport passengers in and out of the park.

All the same, we headed toward Scouts Lookout at fifty-seven hundred feet, which was a nice, easy hike on a well-blazed trail. At the end of it, there were an additional one thousand feet straight up which had to be climbed with hand-held chains securely fastened to some boulders. For that part of the climb, there were six-thousand-foot drops on either side.

Just before Scouts Lookout, I looked for the perfect spot to propose to Paulina. I wanted it to be somewhere she could close her eyes, and where I could set up my phone to record everything. I finally picked out the place and put my plan into action, telling Paulina to close her eyes and not to open them until I said so. As I was adjusting my phone, a fellow hiker offered his assistance, with no idea what he was about to witness. With that, I took a knee and reminded Paulina to keep her eyes closed.

"Baby, I'm not the smartest guy in the world," I began.

"Yes you are!" she interrupted.

"I'm not the richest man in the world," I continued. Again, she replied, "Yes you are!"

"And I'm certainly not the handsomest guy in the world," I said, "but if you would marry me, I'd be the luckiest guy in the world." With that, I presented Paulina the ring as she opened her eyes wide and gave me a huge hug.

"You're my best friend," she said. "Of course I say yes!" Some other hikers had gathered around us and one of the families had a professional camera. When Paulina accepted and we kissed, the entire crowd around us started to applaud. Once again, it felt like the universe was winking at us with its impeccable timing.

When we got to Scout's Lookout, I was considering calling it a day—but without hesitation, Paulina went straight for the first set of chains toward Angels Landing. As I started to voice my concerns, she cut me off.

"Honey, we do CrossFit," she said gently—and of course, I followed her like a lost puppy. When we finally made it to the top, we were looking out at one of the most spectacularly beautiful spots on the entire globe: a panoramic view of Zion, Utah from seven thousand feet up. My proposal had been a huge success. Later that day, when we were on our way out of the park, I reached over to hold her hand. We shared a kiss, and she squeezed my hand in return.

"Seriously," I said, in awe of the world around me. "How did I get so lucky?" She looked at me with a smile that was almost turning into a smirk.

"You did the work," she replied.

PART 3

EIGHT RECOVERY PRINCIPLES FOR BREATHWORK WITH STEPWORK

INTRODUCTION

Twelve Step is the most popular recovery paradigm in the world right now and it has been for a long time, but although it has helped a lot of people, there's often some resistance to following its rules and processes. Even for those who support 12-Step teachings and have used them to get long stretches of sober time, many still struggle to avoid relapses if AA is their only tool.

As I mentioned earlier, I didn't write this book in opposition to AA, though I've known many people who have decided not to continue working a 12-Step program and have still remained sober. Instead, my hope is to supplement the teachings of AA by linking them to the principles of breathwork. More specifically, I want to outline the basic principles of a successful breathwork practice that is oriented toward recovery from addiction and mental illness.

The steps that follow are in a rough order that tries to mirror the stages of an expanding consciousness. In reality, all of these principles apply at all times, in varying degrees of importance, depending on where you are in life. In a sense, the only principles in a relatively fixed place are the first and the last, because any recovery journey has to begin with surrendering the old ways of doing things, and hopefully "ends" with a complete and true sense of spirituality—but even that isn't entirely accurate.

The best way to think of it is in line with the Hero's Journey as outlined by the world-famous writer Joseph Campbell. In his writing he describes the "monomyth," which he says is a structure behind all Western storytelling. In the beginning, an ordinary person is called to an adventure which they initially refuse for any number of reasons: they are either too afraid, or too attached to their world in its current state. Eventually (and often with supernatural aid), they accept the call and cross a threshold, separating themselves from the world they once knew.

For a long time after that, they wander through a confusing, upside-down world full of trials, monsters, lessons and spiritual realizations. They go through darker and harder experiences than they thought possible, and eventually they cross the threshold again, back into the world in which they began, this time with a new understanding from the other side. Now that they've changed, they are masters of both worlds and they're free to live in balance... until they are called to their *next* adventure, and the process begins again.

Campbell's system works literally: it can tell the story of a knight who is recruited to go slay a terrible dragon, but the knight refuses at first because he has a family he loves and he wants to keep safe. A wise man shows him the future if he doesn't go, so the knight embarks on adventure: he does many dangerous things, almost dies, kills the dragon and returns with the dragon's gold. All of that works fine, but on another level, the Hero's Journey should be thought of as a metaphor for the transformation and growth of our consciousness—and the story of addiction and recovery is no different.

At the beginning, our lives are in chaos and a little voice calls on us to make a big change, get sober and clean up our lives. We refuse, because we fear it will be too hard. Usually, addicts experience a glimpse of something greater than themselves that helps them "accept the call" to get sober, whether it's a terrible bottoming-out experience or a sudden moment of peace and clarity that feels spiritual. After breaking with their old ways and crossing the threshold of the normal world into "recovery world," they have to face all kinds of horrible and difficult truths about themselves and their behavior, and at times it feels like the truth might destroy them. But at the end, the addict gains a deeper understanding of themselves and the world, connecting with a spiritual force that is greater than they are. Finally, they can return to the old routines of their life with new strength, able to master their own demons as well as the daily challenges of work and relationships.

Once someone has gone through recovery, they don't necessarily *have* to relapse and return through the cycle. The calls to adventure continue, but ideally, they consist of helping other addicts through the same cycle and remaining sober throughout the process. Eckhart Tolle writes about this idea when he says that once you become awake and conscious as a human being, your job becomes helping others have their own awakenings.

In all, the recovery journey is not a physical trip from Point A to Point B. The moment of true surrender is also deeply spiritual, even if it feels fleeting. To put it simply, don't think of these principles as a checklist to complete or something that has an "end" at all. Instead, it's a set of key ideas that you can incorporate into the rest of your recovery practices, making them an ongoing part of your life.

TESTIMONIAL: MARION'S STORY

Time was frozen. Muffled noises passed through the veil where light and shadow danced. Both sound and light were fading fast as my desire to drink the absent air grew more unbearable.

I was three years old, and I was drowning.

Each endless moment that passed heightened my awareness of water's pressure surrounding my small body.

As I began to fade, I saw a disturbance in the light and shadows around me. A dark figure moved swiftly in my periphery: it was Patrick, my brother, and on that day, my savior. I felt his grasp sweep me up and before I could gather what was happening my head breached the surface and time began to move again.

It was there, on the threshold between death and life, that I became satiated. I took my first fully conscious breath, a massive gasp followed by many shorter ones. As the pitter-patter of my heart slowed and my fear dissolved, my breaths became slower, longer and much more mindful. I held each one with gratitude. They soothed me as a nurturing mother would calm a frightened child.

Many years later, I found myself drowning again, though in a different way. Sunk into heartache, I watched the looming cloud of divorce gliding in my direction, and a sorrowful, lonely rainfall came to fill my once-safe vessel.

The only peace I found was in my yoga practice. After an intense hot vinyasa class, I lay there on my belly, marinating in a puddle of sweat while tears wet my cheeks.

"God, please help me," I whispered softly. "I don't know how to live and feel this pain. Please." Slowly, the students began to rise, gather their things and talk amongst themselves. The mood was cheerful and full of gratitude, yet I remained heavy and numb. Watching them walk toward the exit, I remained immovable until the room was nearly empty. Eventually, I arose, gathered my things and dragged myself to the exit.

The student in front of me didn't notice I was behind her and let the door close in my face. On the door, a flyer read, "Community, Love, Hope and Peace. The time is NOW." I stood looking at the words, thinking I would love to have all of those things. As I kept scanning, I saw that a yoga teacher training was beginning that upcoming fall. I decided to register.

As fall approached, I began training. I had no idea what I was getting myself into, much less any desire to teach. I was only there to deepen my own practice, with those four promised words at the forefront of my mind. In all, the training was not what I expected, but it was everything I needed. It was where I had my second encounter with conscious breath.

My fellow students and I were told to read a variety of literature explaining breath practices, and to personally implement them daily. The Science of Breath by Yogi Ramacharaka was one of our reading assignments, and I particularly appreciated it, as his approach was perfect for a beginning practitioner such as myself.

As time went on, I finally graduated with my 200 RYT Yoga

Teacher Certificate. It was one of the greatest accomplishments of my life, because it was the first time I had decided to prioritize my spiritual growth and emotional health. After I received my certificate, my mentors encouraged me to teach. They all had a certain faith in me that I didn't have in myself.

"You are gifted, and you would be doing a disservice to people if you didn't show up in this way, Marion," one of them said to me. "People need you." I listened to her suggestion, and in the process, I gradually learned how powerful it was to be of service to others.

Eventually, I was selected as one of the top eight yogis in the nation and was gifted the opportunity to practice on stage for the Prime Minister of India and an audience of fifty-five thousand people, at NRG Stadium in Houston, Texas.

During a roughly two-year period, my yoga career took off, and my husband and I attempted to make amends. I figured that one affair over the entire course of our relationship, which had started when we were 14, was maybe not uncommon and not necessarily a reason to end the relationship. I had also become pregnant with our fourth child. After thinking things through, I stayed the course of my healing path, prioritizing my spiritual health as much as I could and attending weekly therapy.

When I was seven months pregnant, I got new information from my best friend of 15 years that shook my entire world: she and my husband had been having an affair. While I was reeling from the news, a practical stranger showed up to my meditation studio and asked to speak to me privately. She had heard through the grapevine what had happened, and she handed me a key.

"This is a key to my house," she said. "There are three bedrooms downstairs and two Pack 'n Play mattresses. No pressure to use the key, but I want you to know you have an escape available that you can use anytime—and promise me you will if you need to." I thanked her and took the key, and with that, she left.

The stress of my circumstances sent me into preterm labor and I ended up in the hospital. I sat alone weeping, terrified my baby would die. The only person who showed up for me during that time was the same mentor who first told me to become a teacher, and who saw strength in me that I didn't know I had. Now, she was reminding me of that strength once more.

I was later discharged and successfully carried the baby to term. He was born healthy and beautiful, which was a much-needed reprieve from my heartache. When he was three months old, I received a picture of a woman, my husband and my baby naked together in my bed. The woman was a stripper my husband had an affair with two years prior. She called me to explain how angry she was that he was cheating on her with a new mistress—and with that call, I grabbed two bags, my four children and the $35 I had. I was ready to use the key.

I filed for divorce shortly after and went into four long years of mediation which left me broken—emotionally, spiritually and financially. In the end, I lost my kids, my spiritual practices, my family, my financial security and my will to live. I had lost everything, and I had nothing left.

I managed to find a way to the Big Island of Hawaii. I had always dreamed of going there, and I hoped it would be a place I could recover and heal. If I was going to be broken and homeless, I figured, I might as well do it in paradise. During that time, the only solace I could find from my daily agony came in the form of a bottle. The instant relief and carelessness that alcohol gave me led to it becoming my only friend.

Coming from a family of addicts, I knew the consequences would eventually catch up to me. Still, I had thoroughly contemplated all possible forms of suicide, and I decided drinking myself to death would be the best way to die.

As my depression worsened, I found myself drowning yet again—this time intentionally, in a bottle. I started getting the shakes, and the reality of my impending death began to set in. I started to question myself: was this really what I wanted?

I decided to go to my favorite cold spring where the honu, Hawaiian sea turtles, go to seek sanctuary from the dangers of the ocean. I sat with the honu in their protected place, crying from the depths of my soul and watching them nurture themselves, wondering how and when I had lost that peaceful version of myself. Feeling completely hopeless and alone, I finally decided to ask for help.

I called a dear friend who I now consider ohana, or family, and he came to my rescue by calling local alcohol treatment facilities. Eventually a man named John shared the name of his facility: Honu House. It was obvious this was part of my divine plan. It was there that I met Nick Terry, the co-owner of the facility, and the man who gracefully led me back to conscious breathwork.

I was terrified when I entered the treatment center, having never been anywhere like it before. Still, I knew I was at the mercy of the universe, with no choice but to trust in what was to come and surrender to the divine plan.

At the beginning of my stay, I sat in the garden crying like a kindergartener on the first day of school. After a few moments, Nick came out of what seemed like thin air to hand me a piece of fresh lavender.

"Breathe this in," he said, before walking away. He spoke my love language and he had a special energy about him. It was the energy of someone who regularly prioritized his own spiritual practice. Because I had known energies like that before, I immediately gave him my innate trust.

Throughout my stay, Nick would lead early morning Wim Hof breathwork practices and meditations, which were pivotal to my healing. Without them, I most likely would not have stuck around. Nick reintroduced me to a practice I had lost, and he held sacred space while I recentered myself in my spiritual healing.

As a result of his program, I now have a beautiful life. I have systems in place to keep my sobriety and spirituality intact, and I recognize that without them I become lost and ultimately drown. Breathwork is a cornerstone for me and will always remain a priority—and I will forever be grateful to Nick and the Honu House staff for showing me the way.

1

SURRENDER

One thing almost all addicts have in common is that they realize they have a problem long before they actually get sober or find recovery. Part of the issue is that addiction often starts as a solution for another, bigger problem—whether it's childhood trauma, anxiety, or disconnection. For a while, drugs and alcohol can cover up a problem by making the user feel better or taking stress away, but over time, those effects wear off.

As the drugs and alcohol get less effective and addiction starts to set in, one of the hardest things for an addict to admit is that *they were wrong*. Their way of doing things steered them in the wrong direction and they don't know how to get out of it. Since admitting their mistake and facing it head-on is so painful, many addicts cling to their bad habits, preventing them from ever fully recovering.

In the 12 Steps, the first few steps are to admit you are powerless over alcohol and drugs, to believe in a Higher Power that can restore your sanity, and to turn your life over to God . Taken together, these first steps are essentially asking addicts to surrender.

In my own life, I spent many years knowing I had a problem but not being able to solve it. For a little over five years, I circled the perimeter of recovery, always with one eye on the door. In Chapter Five of the Big Book of AA, it says, "half measures availed us nothing," which was certainly the case with me. I'd get a little bit of time sober and a little bit of abstinence, but I never fully surrendered my old ideas and ways of behaving in favor of permanent, long-term sobriety. Although I wasn't aware of it at the time, I was half-surrendered and half-committed, so I never fully got better.

It's a lonely world when you are half-surrendered. You know you can't drink or use like "normal people," whoever they are, but you're also not committing to do what it takes to give up drugs and alcohol and find a better path. Equally dark and lonely is the experience of maintaining some periods of abstinence through treatment and going to 12-Step meetings, but not experiencing any of the happiness, joy and freedom people talk about as a result.

When I was getting sober, I went to four inpatient residential treatment programs and several outpatient programs, so I attended a lot of recovery meetings. During that time, I heard people say things like:

"Something happened."

"Something shifted."

"I believe that's when God happened."

"That's when surrender happened."

"That's when the universal spirit happened."

"I believe that's when recovery happened for me."

My struggle for many years, both before I got sober and in early sobriety, was that I couldn't really relate to those experiences. When I finally did surrender, of course my life changed dramatically, but it didn't happen the way I expected. When I was first getting sober, I knew I'd made a ton of mistakes and had to get better, but for a long time I didn't feel any magical presence of a Higher Power guiding me—or if I did, it was only a glimmer, something that could be written off as a coincidence.

To me, the real surrender was the realization that sobriety and recovery weren't only—or even primarily—about not drinking or using drugs. More than that, it was about surrendering my old identity, my old ways of doing and thinking about things, and not trying to get them back. Without complete surrender, I knew true change wouldn't be possible—but the thing about surrender is, there's no real way to know if you've done it yet until you finally do. Once I actually surrendered, something *did* shift. My thoughts started to change, and so did the way I behaved. In essence, I eventually had enough experiences to make sense of what a Higher Power meant to me and lean into it—but that process took many years, and many addicts don't have years to wait around for that realization.

What's often missing from 12-Step groups at the very beginning are supporting tools and usable strategies to help addicts in early recovery achieve their goals. On some level, a person has to want to do those things for themselves. But at the same time, it's possible to work with your body to change how you think and feel, easing yourself into a state of surrender. That's a lot more practical than just stopping all drug use and praying for a change. Though AA recommends prayer and meditation, prayer often feels very strange to people who aren't used to it, and meditation is often too complicated and difficult to get into, even for people who have a lot of sober time.

AA claims that the beginning of recovery and the solution to addiction is a spiritual awakening, or a shift in consciousness. If addiction is an obsession or compulsion and you're looking to change it, you need a shift in consciousness. So, how do you create that? In my case, if I had been exposed to the power of breathwork much earlier in my recovery journey, I think I would have found surrender much faster. Fortunately, people who are new to sobriety are free to take advantage of what I didn't know.

The process of surrendering takes a lot of self-reflection, and that can be done through journaling, prayer, meditation, exercise, yoga, or art. All of these are effective outlets, but what often doesn't get said is that intense self-reflection can be dangerous and triggering for some people. It's important work, but it stirs up powerful negative emotions that can lead to relapses if you're not careful. When I work with clients in recovery, I recommend that they focus on their diet and some kind of exercise routine to help regulate their bodies and emotions, but that can take time to be fully effective. The good thing about breathwork is that it's fast-acting, low effort and effective, and it can take us out of a triggered state to a calm one very quickly.

While it's important to surrender, it's also necessary to have tools at your disposal to deal with everything you're stirring up in the process. To that end, it's a good idea to make breathwork a part of your routine in addition to everything else you're doing for recovery. Start your morning with a quick breathing exercise (either energizing or relaxing, depending on what you need), and then do a quick recharge around lunchtime. If you suddenly feel overwhelmed or tempted to drink or use, do all the things you would normally do like calling your sponsor— and remember you can *also* do a relaxing breathwork exercise to return your emotional state to normal.

Doing the right kind of breathwork while you're in a heightened state can be a very powerful tool for transformation and surrender. Oftentimes when we have a huge emotional spike, a lot of the spiraling thoughts we have are ego-driven, anxious and angry. They're usually totally ungrounded and untrue, but they come on so quickly and automatically that they can carry us away. By doing breathwork right as those thoughts are happening, an amazing thing can happen. Sometimes, we feel ourselves sinking deeper into our emotions— almost like we're passing *through* the thought and going right to the feeling. Sitting in our feelings can also be uncomfortable, but if we focus on the in-and-out of the breath, we can actually *pass* those feelings and return to normal. It's an interesting way to illustrate the concept of surrender: through our breath, we are surrendering our trapped emotions back into the world around us, almost like the breath is shoveling them out .

Though it will still take repetition and practice, along with the help of all the other recovery interventions, breathwork is a healthy way to release emotions that have been stopped up for too long. It can help us get our minds in touch with our hearts and spirits, which is where true surrender happens. And that's what makes change and recovery possible.

If you've been tortured by the diseases of addiction, alcoholism, codependency, depression, anxiety, panic and fear, there is a way out—and in my experience, surrender is the imperative first movement towards freedom, happiness and connection. In the AA rooms, many of us will hear the term HOW, which stands for Honesty, Open-mindedness and Willingness. But speaking personally, HOW should be SHOW, because Surrender needs to come first.

2

CLARITY

If the first step of recovery is surrender—in other words, to admit that we were wrong about how we were doing things and how we understood ourselves and the world—then the next step is to start learning and embracing how things *actually are*. And when you've been living a life of lies, dishonesty and illusion for a very long time, that's not such an easy task. Baked into both the first few Steps and the concept of surrender in general is that by turning away from what's not true, we'll turn towards what *is* true. It roughly corresponds to what alcoholics sometimes call "a moment of clarity," because clarity is what's needed to move forward in recovery.

Clarity doesn't necessarily mean that there's one objectively correct way to do everything. It's not about applying one moral code to all kinds of behavior. Instead, it's about dealing with the reality of things as they are, without judgment or denial. On one level, clarity can mean admitting that hiding alcohol and drugs from your family is a bad idea, or realizing that addiction *does* affect your ability to be a good parent or hold down a job. On another level, clarity can be much more subjective. It can mean admitting that you *don't* forgive your parents for their mistakes yet, even though you've been saying for years that you did. Alternatively, maybe clarity means admitting that a grudge you've been holding for years was actually an overreaction, and you need to apologize and make things right.

Finally, on a more religious or spiritual level, clarity means starting to dissolve some of the categories we use to divide and judge things, coming to the understanding that everything is connected. It means starting to realize that the difference between "us" and "them" is mostly in our minds, and that we're not the center of the universe but just another interconnected part of it. Learning to look at things this way helps us in recovery because it expands our consciousness, whereas addiction tends to narrow our perspective until we can't even see past ourselves. It builds on surrendering, because once we have clarity about how things actually are, we can finally begin to understand what we need to do to live in harmony.

Clarity is less about what's right and wrong than it is about the world being run by laws, even if they're invisible to us. When we break certain laws or guidelines, there are always consequences—even if they take a while to catch up to us. One example is the fact that the more we use drugs, the less benefit and the more harm will come from them. Another is that the more we manipulate people and lie, the fewer people we'll have left around us until we're completely alone. A lot of these principles are discussed in 12-Step programs, but they also apply to breathwork and our understanding of it—even down to the basic meaning of the word "breath" across many different languages.

In many ancient cultures, "breath," "spirit" and "soul" share the same word or meaning. *Pneuma* (πνεῦμα) is an ancient Greek word for "breath," though it also means "spirit" or "soul" when used in a religious context. In the Hawaiian language and culture, the word *aloha* means "the breath of life" or the "breath of God," depending on the interpretation (broken down, *alo* means "the embodiment of God or life" and *ha* means "breath"). When native Hawaiians greet each other, it's customary that they touch foreheads and share an exhalation: *ha*.

In India's Hindu philosophy—including yoga, medicine and martial arts—there is a central concept of *prana* (प्राण), a Sanskrit word meaning life force or vital energy. It was also a basic ancient theory of reality, similar to atomic theory: prana was said to permeate reality on all levels, including both living beings and inanimate objects. In China, concept of *chi* emerged about three thousand years ago. The Chinese believed that the body contained channels that functioned like power lines between different organs, letting chi flow between them. If you look into Native American tribes like the Mohawk, Oneida, Onondaga, Cayuga, Seneca and Iroquois, you'll see similar themes.

Throughout a multitude of cultures, the basic words and expressions for breath are synonymous with God, spirit and soul. Of course, I can't *prove* that this coincidence means that breathwork is a direct line to God or a direct pathway to your spirituality. In my experience though, breathwork has been so helpful that it might as well be. Countless people have reported how breathwork has made them think more clearly, have realizations and feel more spiritually connected to themselves and the world around them. Many people have also said this about meditation, which is why so many different meditation practices emphasize breath control, sometimes calling breath "the leash" of the mind.

In some sense, surrendering and getting a true sense of spirituality is similar to the concept of being "enlightened" or awakened. In his teachings, Eckhart Tolle describes enlightenment as a general condition of spending more time in consciousness than time lost in "ruminating thought." To put it in AA terms, it's the "ruminating thought" of our own petty identities that we need to surrender and give up. We use drugs and alcohol to silence our thoughts, but the cycle of having the thoughts, then using drugs to silence them leaves us powerless. Fortunately, having the clarity to admit that and accept it returns some of our power back to us.

As I mentioned before, the recovery community currently puts a lot of emphasis on meditation as a way to clear our minds of ruminating thoughts, along with surrendering to a Higher Power with prayer, even if we don't understand it. I think meditation is amazing, but it can often be too advanced for someone in early recovery. I tried meditating throughout the years while I was sober, but it wasn't until I had a daily breathwork practice that I could actually stick to meditation and unlock all of its benefits. For the last few years, I've been keeping a daily breathwork practice, and the benefits I've experienced have been incredible.

3

HONESTY

The first two of the 12 Steps are about letting go of our own will and surrendering to a new way of doing things. As addicts transition into Step Three and beyond, the process takes a turn. If the initial stages are about admitting our own wrongs and recognizing the way things really are, the next stages are about living in alignment with that new reality. In short, it's about learning to be honest.

In my own life, I always prided myself on "keeping it real" throughout my younger years—even though in reality, my entire life was a lie. My sponsor Phil brought this to my attention when I was doing my Fourth Step work.

"What role has dishonesty played in your life?" he asked me. I told him that I lied a lot about my drinking and using, but that I was a fairly honest person overall. He didn't accept that, and challenged me to go back through my life and find other times I was dishonest before I picked up a drink or a drug. As I started reflecting, the journey I went on was mind-blowing. I'd been telling lies and half-truths since I was five years old.

My dishonesty began with keeping secrets, and it was the

root of what I call my "spiritual malady." I believe that the human spirit has a deep desire to have an open dialogue and that it dislikes secrecy. We want to have transparency at the deepest level. Our souls and spirits yearn for it, and part of our sickness as alcoholics and addicts lies in keeping secrets and not being our authentic selves. Part of the sickness is not being able to tell the entire story of things and not being able to be vulnerable and courageous. For me, it meant that I started making things up as a little kid. Throughout my adolescence and in my young adulthood, the alternative stories I made up about my life created the fabric of my existence. I was living a double life even before I touched drugs and alcohol.

When I tell my recovery story , I start with my first memories of being dishonest. It's a very important piece of my recovery puzzle. What was it about my life that felt so inadequate, so fundamentally wrong that I had to create another identity? When I finally started to look at those things, I began to understand what had been happening in my childhood household at a much deeper level—including all the dysfunction, trauma, abandonment and toxicity.

Though I hadn't realized it, my dishonesty was a symptom of a few underlying causes. As early as I could remember, I was constantly around people using drugs, and they were often violent and abusive. It wasn't something that I felt I could share openly with the rest of the world, and doing so would've made me feel even less safe than I already was. Even though the adults in my life never explicitly told me not to talk about all that dysfunction, it was still something that I felt was communicated intuitively ever since I was young.

The recurring theme of my life throughout early childhood was separation. I felt different and alone, and I didn't know where I fit in the grand scheme of things. When I discovered drugs and alcohol, they gave me a feeling of belonging and connection that I'd been looking for—even if it was artificial, didn't last and eventually started to destroy everything important in my life.

It was both interesting and not totally surprising to discover in recovery that my dishonesty wasn't connected to my drug addiction or alcoholism. It predated both, and I wasn't aware of the impact it was having on who I was. As I made a personal inventory, I saw that lying, cheating and manipulating were a big part of all my relationships. I wasn't comfortable in my own skin. I wasn't comfortable in the environment in which I was raised. I wasn't comfortable on this planet. After my spiritual shift in early sobriety, it became abundantly clear to me that I couldn't lie any longer. By making that change, I started to develop a personal moral compass. Had I known about it earlier, I believe that breathwork would've helped me make that shift even sooner.

There are many different kinds of breathing exercises, but regardless of which one you do, each of them is fundamentally *honest*. The simple act of breathing in an intentional way puts you directly in touch with your body and what's *really* going on inside it. This can be as simple as doing a breathing awareness exercise to check whether you're breathing deeply or shallowly, if you're carrying any tension, or if you're truly at ease. In more stimulating breathing exercises like the Wim Hof or Tummo methods, the first few times you do it might bring the anxiety or anger you've been hiding to the surface in a sudden rush, and breathing through it will let it pass. On the more extreme end, doing a longer session of clarity breathwork can stir up very deep trauma that you might not even be aware of and help release it (though I wouldn't recommend this to beginners, especially not without supervision).

Other activities like exercise, meditation, journaling and yoga can all help to clear the mind and create space for reflection, but I've found that breathwork is the perfect complement to each of them, and it's often missing from peoples' routines. All four of those activities are great, but each one can be challenging for someone early in recovery. I always highly recommend exercise, but it can take practice for some people not to feel angry or insecure at the gym. Likewise, meditation, journaling and yoga can require a lot of patience and attention to reap their full benefits, and addicts in early recovery don't always have those things. Breathwork, on the other hand, can be done in as few as 10 minutes and it has an almost immediate beneficial effect. We often think of honesty as an abstract intellectual concept, but breathwork will show you that honesty actually starts in our bodies in a very real and physical way.

Over time, I've realized that honesty is the most important part of my new way of living. Being honest with other people—and most importantly, being honest with myself when it comes to doing the right-but-uncomfortable thing—has been the bedrock of my recovery. In addition to breathwork, one technique I recommend is simple: *tell on yourself* if you notice you're being dishonest, even if it's strange or awkward.

In the first few years of my recovery, I would tell someone a story before suddenly realizing that I'd actually just lied again without noticing—and then another lie would follow. Whenever I caught myself doing it, I had to tattle on myself. One of my favorite acronyms is DENIAL— Don't Even Notice I Am Lying. Fortunately, I finally started to notice and to care.

"That's not how the story went," I would say. "That's not exactly how it happened. What I said just now wasn't the truth; I apologize. I was being dishonest, but I'm working on becoming a better person." The look on people's faces was priceless. People in recovery understood what I was going through, but others would be confused, or else they'd dismiss what I was saying as "not a big deal." For me, it was an imperative piece of my spiritual recovery, and I couldn't compromise on it. Honesty is the first agreement in Don Miguel Ruiz's timeless classic *The Four Agreements* for a reason, and I can testify that it has the power to completely transform your life!

If you're reading this book and have been struggling with addiction in any form, I challenge you to look all the way back and ask: what lies have I been telling myself? What lies have I been telling others? What stories have I been holding onto that aren't true? Write them all down, look at them and see if you can discern what were the root causes of your dishonesty. To aid in your process, adopt a breathwork practice to make being centered and honest in your body a lifelong habit.

TESTIMONIAL: JEFF'S STORY

I was born and raised in Staten Island, New York. I was a good kid, loved my family, had many friends and a great love for animals. My dad was a police officer, and my mom did her best to raise me and my older sister, Carolyn. My immediate family was warm and close, and I received a lot of love growing up, especially around the holidays. I attended Catholic school as a child and participated in sports and school activities. There were many family vacations to Florida and upstate New York, and my father tried to expose me to as many fun activities as he could. I think I learned to snow and waterski before I learned the alphabet! My sister was a swimmer and I was a soccer star, and we'd both fight over the Staten Island Advance on Sunday mornings to see who made the sports section of the local paper.

Although my earliest memories were happy, it didn't take long before I noticed the dark side of my environment. In the fourth grade, my mother thought I could get a better education at a larger school in a larger neighborhood, so I transferred to Blessed Sacrament. I was the new kid on the block with a lot to prove, and if you were "uncool," you were cast out.

129

The kind, quieter types were picked-on, bullied and often humiliated. The uncool kid were beaten up or jumped, often two or three against one. As the threats of physical violence and emotional abuse became part of my social life, I quickly tried to become "cool," fitting this new mask as best I could. I studied the behavior of others and emulated it, quickly becoming a chameleon. In 5th grade, I started drinking, smoking cigarettes and experimenting with marijuana, which subsequently led to various forms of lying to conceal my behavior and whereabouts.

I spent hours practicing my father's signature so I could self-authorize my frequent absences and started to falsify my report cards and school documents. To go above and beyond in proving my "cool" status, I decided to pack my father's antique gun in my backpack one day and off to school I went. I had no experience using a gun and knew I was making a really bad decision. I was carrying a deadly weapon into a crowded school and was completely terrified. I knew I had gone too far.

In just a few hours, I was caught. That incident, and many others like it, changed the course of my life forever.

The shame and anxiety of being suspended and eventually expelled from school was traumatic, and it shifted my personality. My behavior departed from the good-natured values I had carried as long as I could remember. My thoughts now were scattered, and I felt as though a grenade had exploded next to my head. With no real evidence, I imagined my family hated me. I felt abandoned, so I shut down and assumed the identity of the black sheep. I began running away from home and sneaking out at night to drink and smoke pot.

Soon, lying, cheating and stealing all became part of my daily life until I got in enough trouble that my mother had no choice but to have me transfer schools again. In the middle of the 7th grade, I transferred to IS 61, known as a "cool" school because accountability for attendance was not one of the school's strong points.

On my first day, I was greeted by several of my new class-mates who had heard rumors about me. Instead of being shamed for what I had done, they celebrated me! From day one, I was given the identity of the crazy, tough guy who brought a gun to school. The attention was intoxicating, especially from the girls —so I ran with it. The trend carried throughout high school, and soon I started to feel like a rock star.

In the mid-80's in Staten Island, cocaine was popular and bars allowed access to minors. If you could reach the bar, you were allowed to drink—and so I did, which was like pouring gasoline on an already-raging dumpster fire. By senior year of high school, I was a mess. I rarely attended class, I would try to sleep all day, my mother was a wreck, my sister was terrified and angry and my behavior was out of control. Around the same time, my father got promoted and became a federal narcotics officer in New York City, and I represented everything he stood against. Eventually, it culminated in an intervention.

My father presented me with three options: go to college outside of New York State, join the US Navy or back my bags and go. The next day, he took me to the Navy Recruiting station, and off I went to San Diego for boot camp.

The Navy served me well. I earned a position as a radioman in the communications department, and I loved it. With some structure, I was able to clean up, grow up, learn a lot of skills and excel. Within months, I was in the fleet headed to the Persian Gulf on an amphibious assault ship loaded with 1500 Marines as part of Operation Desert Storm. In my four years of service, we completed four major deployments.

I learned a bit about cross addiction in the Navy, although I didn't know it at the time. Since there was no access to drugs or alcohol while out to sea, I developed a sufficient substitute: over-

working. Being a communication specialist with a top-secret security clearance, I saw that I could become highly valued and highly praised by high-ranking officers because we controlled all the communications on the ship.

Though it may go without saying, the ability for the ship to communicate with mobile SEAL teams and Marine units conducting air, sea and land operations in a hostile territory is crucial. I knew getting to the top of that communication hierarchy was going to take a lot of effort, and I was ready to put it in. Before long, I was starting to get noticed—even if it required working 18 hours a day sometimes.

My lucky break came on deployment, when my predecessors who taught me everything I knew about communications all discharged around the same time and left me with all their knowledge and responsibilities. My hard work finally paid off and in great measure. Now, I was the man! The feeling was electric. Once again, I felt celebrated, valued and popular with the other officers all the way to the top, as they depended on me for their vital communication systems.

The longer and harder I worked, the more praise and recognition I received, and soon it became another reinforced addiction. I noticed that the moment we pulled into port and let me off the ship, my drinking got me in trouble. Fortunately, most, if not all, of the consequences were mitigated or excused because of the unique circumstances on the ship—which I later learned was just about the worst thing that could happen to an alcoholic.

After seeing how successful I was in the military, when my time was up, I decided to discharge from the Navy to pursue financial fortunes. Though I was unaware of it at the time, I was going to bring all my untreated trauma and work-addiction tendencies with me into civilian life.

For the next four years, I worked my ass off trying to stay one step ahead of my addiction and alcoholism. I was able to land a *promising job in the field of information technology, and once again started working long hours to chase my dreams of financial success. Soon, I was hired as Director of Information Technology at a major fiber optics company in Sorrento Valley, San Diego. The industry was booming, and I was given a terrific salary with stock options and an unlimited budget with the go-ahead to hire an entire team of technicians to build an IT Department. I even made the cover of Information Security magazine!*

At the same time, my disease was equally hard at work. During the same period that I was excelling in the office, I had two DUIs, multiple broken relationships and was arrested multiple times for driving without a license. I was living a double life: IT Director by day and cocaine-fueled drunken lunatic by night. But once again, I worked so hard and made myself so valuable to the company that all of my absences and indiscretions were excused. The team I hired were all financially dependent on me, so they became great enablers—up to the moment that two police officers arrived at my work and apprehended me for an outstanding warrant, which was not one of my proudest moments.

In late 2004, I was informed that the company would be sold and that my duty was to support the CFO in laying off most of the employees, including my own team. When that was done, I would receive a hefty bonus and a severance package on my way out. I was set! Once the job was done and it was time for me to receive my bonus, the CEO sat down with me with a check in his hand. "I know about your condition," he said. "You have a very serious illness. And without treatment, this check in my hand will end up killing you."

I couldn't believe what I was hearing as he explained to me that he had the same illness, but that he was in recovery and had been sober for 30 years. As he described the insanity of his own experiences with alcoholism, I was floored. At that moment, I was no longer alone. There was hope. I immediately agreed to let him hold my check while I went to find help. Soon after, I checked into the VA hospital. From there, I was admitted to a nine-month, social model recovery home in South Park, San Diego, where I fell in love with the idea of helping others to heal myself.

For the first time in my life, I surrendered all my grand plans and great ideas because the very best of them landed me in a glorified homeless shelter for alcoholic men. That was the result of my best game! While I was in treatment, I decided to change careers and join the field of drug and alcohol treatment. I completed San Diego City College's AODS program and was asked to teach drug and alcohol education, a voluntary commitment I held for the next six years.

I took suggestions, got a sponsor, went to meetings regularly, started sponsoring other men and watched as my life became amazing. The more active I was in my recovery program, the more the promises of what sobriety held came true. I got a job at a psychiatric therapeutic community and loved it. The money wasn't great but, as I had learned from the Navy and my other jobs, I knew hard work would pay off. In fact, I was determined to open my own center one day!

For the next six years, I worked hard and learned everything I could and quickly rose through the ranks. I became a staff supervisor, then housing director, then director of operations. Later, I became my facility's lead interventionist, and started traveling from city to city multiple times per week. At the same time, the owners partnered with me to let me open my own independent living home. All of it was great except for one small problem: the work I was doing for my own recovery was faltering, and was almost a distant memory.

After taking on so many duties, I had stopped going to meet-

ings and doing the things I'd learned in treatment. I was stressed and fatigued beyond comprehension, and began to develop superior oblique myokymia, a condition where the muscle that holds the eye in place becomes strained and distorts vision. The condition was intermittent and could fluctuate in intensity, sometimes making it unbearable to read, think or focus. It added to my mental fatigue, depression and fogginess, though I didn't know it would plague me for the next 10 years.

At about five years of sobriety, while leaving the office, I remembered that there was Adderall in one of the medication cabinets I had access to. Without hesitation, I stole it—and I was off and running. That one decision triggered a series of methamphetamine and alcohol relapses that resulted in losing my job, my dignity, my sanity and almost my life. Despite having previous experience with recovery, the knowledge did nothing. I could not stop of my own willpower, no matter how painful the consequences of my actions were becoming. My addiction raged and brought me to the darkest places. Soon, I knew I had only two options left: suicide or recovery. The latter seemed elusive, as I had never felt so completely and desperately powerless.

Miraculously, I had a small window of pain, suffering and humiliation where my addiction relented, coupled with me having enough strength and clarity to ask for help. Once again, I sobered up, completed treatment and got back on the horse. Within months, I was mostly healthy again, other than my superior oblique myokymia—which on most days was so uncomfortable that it was hard to see the point in even existing.For years I saw doctors for my condition but none of their recommendations or medications worked. It was very difficult to isolate and diagnose, and with no medical solution, I tried to tolerate it as best I could.

I was instrumental in opening a detox center in Ramona,

California and helped open several other treatment centers and sober living homes. It all led to partnering with Dr. Mark Melden to open our own facility, Crownview Co-Occurring Institute, in 2004. Since we had no employees and no money other than Mark's savings, I had no choice but to live with clients for the first two years. Once again, I was working around the clock. Though our program began in National City, California as a small psychiatric residential treatment program, over the next nine years, it flourished.

Throughout the early years of my recovery, I struggled with sobriety. I saw countless therapists to help me through, but the treatments didn't stick. I would always start off well, but over time, I ended up with the same result. I started to believe there was something uniquely wrong with me and that recovery would never work. I was losing hope in myself, as were my friends and co-workers, until I met Nick Terry through a friend in 2021.

I learned Nick was in Hawaii, and he was doing something different. This piqued my interest, because I knew I had tried just about everything else. When I spoke to Nick, he started telling me about breathwork, and he even did a small demonstration over the phone. I decided to come to Maui to meet him, and the first time I tried breathwork in person, I had a very strange sensation. By the third round, I was overwhelmed by all the grief and sadness that came rushing to the surface. It was a sudden and unexpected release of emotion—and it must have been contagious, because when I opened my eyes, all six of the other people I had been doing breathwork with were all crying as well!

Over the next two weeks, I started the day with three rounds of breathwork. One day, I noticed I had not had any symptoms of superior oblique myokymia. A condition I'd suffered from for 10 years, now resolved from breathing! Could it be true? I inadvertently tested the theory when I returned to San Diego for work, where I learned again how much easier it was to start the day with coffee, fear, worry and excessive over-thinking rather than a spiritual practice that required a little time, commitment and energy. The very name, breathwork, implies effort.

I fell off my breathwork routine and, in about seven days, my symptoms returned. Seeing this, I immediately reprioritized it, and my symptoms haven't returned since. That was 14 months ago.

Breathwork helps me cope with a host of uncomfortable emotions like resentment, fear, anxiety and depression. When I find myself tangled up with life, I pause and breathe a few rounds. I always feel better and clearer after a good session, and I believe in its efficacy so much that I've also worked into the curriculum at Crownview.

In addition to breathwork, Nick Terry introduced me to a few other modalities that have changed my life, including cold water emersion therapy. When I got to the point where I could tolerate two minutes or so, I started to feel the benefits and experienced a profound natural high, followed by a lasting sense of well-being, significant increase of energy and better sleep. After some research, I learned that these experiences were backed by science along with other benefits, one of which was mental resilience.

It is evident that people suffering from addiction don't do well with feeling uncomfortable. Cold water immersion therapy, in my experience, trains the brain how to sit in discomfort and helps build resilience. I have since converted by garage into a small wellness center with a cold plunge tub as a central part of the design.

Finally, Nick also introduced me to IFS therapy to treat my early childhood trauma, EMDR for my military and civilian trauma and mindfulness and meditation practices that I've incorporated into daily practices and a new way of life. He has emphasized to me that the only way I will remain sober is if I fully integrate myself into a community of recovery, spirituality and service to others and remain consistent in a daily routine.

I have followed Nick's advice and made all these components part of my routine. As a result, I now have 14 months of sobriety and a full and wonderful life—better than I could have ever planned myself.

4

COURAGE

Reflecting on your mistakes, admitting you were wrong, seeking help and changing your behavior are all huge steps on the road to recovery. Celebrate them! Each one is its own little victory. Still, as hard as it is to get started, it's just as hard to keep going when you're in the middle and don't know what's coming next.

Between Steps Four to Nine is where the deep recovery work happens and we get a better understanding of the problems that were driving our addiction in the first place. We need to enter that stage with a grounded sense of honesty about the work we have to do, because we know it will include facing difficult emotions and remembering things we'd rather forget. Once we're at that point in the process, the crucial thing we need is the courage to see it through.

Courage is the spiritual principle behind Step Four in the 12 Steps: the inventory process. I had been in and out of meetings and treatment centers for about five years before I had the willingness and courage to actually go through Step Four myself. The word "courage" is derived from a Latin word which means "to tell the entire story from the heart." How appropriate, because telling our stories wholeheartedly is exactly what Step Four requires.

Another way to think of courage is that it's the ability to experience fear and to do what we're afraid of anyway. That process becomes a little easier if we get a better understanding of what fear is in the first place. Personally, my favorite way to define fear is with the acronym False Evidence Appearing Real. My first great fear in sobriety was that I would never be able to stay sober or be a good father, that I was going to live in prison or die a drug addicted, alcoholic death. I was never going to have a career, a meaningful relationship or a home of my own. I was never going to get married or have my own business. Of course, if I let my mind run wild with those thoughts without pausing to examine them, they might easily get control over me. But by using the right tools—including breathwork, exercise, 12-Step principles, spiritual reading, meditation and more—I was able to poke holes in my fears and distance myself from them.

Before the Covid epidemic (and certainly during it), many of us were stressed-out to the max. We've been living in fear, anxiety and depression, and a lot of those symptoms have been taking root in our bodies in the form of a tight neck and shoulders, a clenched jaw, shallow breathing and insomnia. Some of the causes of these symptoms include caffeine, stimulants like Adderall, too much time on social media and the never-ending negativity of the 24-hour news cycle (which can become consuming and addictive in itself). So many of us are being governed and dictated by these powerful cycles of stress, fear and tension, and we need to break free from them. Breathwork and meditation are a great way to do that.

Breathwork is an easy way to get back in touch with our bodies and away from distressing influences in our environment. It can create a space for us to return to center, and see our problems and fears as separate from ourselves. In reality, fears are just another kind of thoughtform. They are separate from our truest self, which is the observer that watches our thoughts. Just as I learned from doing breathwork, reading the work of Eckhart Tolle and attending a quepasana retreat, *we are not our thoughts.* This means that we are not our fears either, even if they can still play a useful role in our lives.

When we see our fears clearly, we perceive that they are actually indicators of the things we love and hold dear. They're a reminder of the things we don't want to lose and we want to protect, but that's all that they should be. They can be quiet passengers, but we don't want to let them hold the steering wheel. On some level, courage comes from how well we can tap into our sense of love and purpose. It means having hard conversations and doing the "right" thing for ourselves and the people we care about, because our love outweighs whatever resistance we have. Breathwork isn't always necessary to be courageous when it matters most, but as a practice, it can help us connect to ourselves and our sense of love and purpose— which is where all courage comes from. When it comes to doing the internal recovery work and fighting through our anxiety and resistance, breathwork is a useful way to boost our courage and help us see things through.

The point of the inventory is not to morbidly reflect on yourself or beat yourself up too much. For me, the goal was to get a clear picture of my wrongs, and what values and character flaws I needed to change in order to transform. The beautiful part of this step was that it was painful—a beautiful pain. As I went through the inventory process and got honest with myself, I finally had the courage to walk the path I was supposed to, to go back and look at my defects of character that were the real roots of my issues.

When I take other people through this same process today,

I look back at my old list of fears and I see that seven years later, none of them has come true. I've never been homeless; in fact, I'm a homeowner now. I'm a great father, and my youngest daughter has lived with me full-time now for five years. I have a meaningful, wonderful relationship that's going to be a marriage someday soon. Though all of the fears I listed were extremely real at the time, none of them has materialized because I've continued this process.

Without completing the inventory process, I could never have asked a spiritual power to remove my defects of character. It was imperative for me to see every resentment, fear and harm done to others clearly, so I could ask my spiritual power to remove them. At the very least, that spiritual power made me aware of them all so that I could change my behavior. The inventory also gave me a list of people to make amends to, people I would have to meet face-to-face to admit that I was wrong and ask what I could do to make things right. That's what I did, and it's what all of us in long-term recovery are called to do.

5

VULNERABILITY

Once we recognize how important courage is to recovery, we tend to think of it in stereotypical ways. We think that courage means being big, brave, strong and powerful, but that's not exactly right. In many cases, having a lot of outer strength, rudeness or defensiveness is actually a way of distracting people from our *lack* of courage. In other situations, courage definitely looks big and heroic, but the root of all real courage is recognizing and admitting that we have things we want to protect because we love them. If we don't care about anything or love anyone (including ourselves), it's hard to be courageous because our "courage" doesn't really *mean* anything. For it to work the way it's supposed to, we need the courage to be vulnerable first.

Brené Brown has a lot to say about why vulnerability is courageous. In her work, she explains that vulnerability is a crucial piece of living a wholehearted life, and that shame is one of the biggest things that gets in the way of expressing it. Her message has special importance to addicts, because shame suffocates most addicts and alcoholics. The cure for that shame, according to Brown, is excruciating vulnerability—being all-the-way seen, no matter the cost.

Though I may sound like a broken record, daily breathwork and meditation have been a crucial part of helping me stay in touch with my vulnerability and use it for long-term recovery. When doing these practices, it's impossible to stay trapped in our thoughts about how we appear to others, or why we fail because of things that happened long in the past. Instead, breathwork brings us into the present moment where everything happens now. Negative thoughts are what Eckhart Tolle would call "emotional pain bodies," as they're thoughtforms that come together to form a kind of energetic template that takes over our *real* body any time we start thinking about them. In order for me to let go of those emotional pain bodies and rewrite my story, I had to begin by doing a full inventory to see where the negative thoughts were coming from. Then, I had to have the vulnerability to let those things pass through me without trying to cling to them.

It's easy to think of vulnerability in the abstract, but I don't think there are many better ways of creating real, physical vulnerability than through breathwork. On the physical level, breathwork and meditation require us to lower our defenses and open our awareness. We release the tension in our bodies and stop trying to physically defend ourselves from attacks. While doing this can be scary, it also signals to our bodies that it's *okay* to release stress because nothing bad will happen to us. The more we practice, the more our bodies will learn that we don't have to look over our shoulders all the time, and the more our anxiety will dissipate.

Breathwork is a very real way of creating and feeling emotional vulnerability—and it's a direct product of our physical vulnerability. There's a famous saying you might have heard that "emotion follows motion." What it means is that we

can guide our emotions by changing our bodies' physical move-
ments. For example, if we're feeling down and low energy, one
of the best things we can do is exercise, even if it's the last thing
we want to do. It's a bit of a paradox, but spending energy actually *gives* us more energy, rather than draining our reserves.
There's a similar relationship that happens between the physical state of our bodies and what our bodies *allow us* to feel at
any given moment.

If we're walking around with extreme tension and nervousness, it's a signal that we're not ready to be calm and do any
heavy, emotional work that might open us to an attack. That
tension is connected to our "fight, flight or freeze" response, and
it explains why sometimes we want to spring into action, while
other times we want to collapse and numb out. Most of the
time, these fight or flight signals happen automatically, but our
body can set them up in maladaptive ways. For example, if we
had an extremely abusive childhood, we will be in an activated
fight, flight or freeze a lot more than someone who didn't—and
often in situations when we don't need to be. Fortunately,
breathwork can help us take back control of these automatic
processes.

Breathing is governed by our autonomic nervous system.
We breathe without thinking, just as we blink and digest food.
Even so, breathing is different from digestion in that we can still
control our breathing patterns if we actively pay attention to
them. When we do so, we can shift two primary parts of our
nervous system. The first is the sympathetic nervous system,
which is responsible for our fight, flight, freeze or fawn
responses that produce fear and anxiety: I sometimes call these
our "relapse and remorse" system. The second part we can shift
is the parasympathetic nervous system, which is responsible for
our "rest and digest" mode and our ability to relax: I think of

this as our "healthy trauma response and relapse prevention" system.

Though all of this is somewhat intuitive, it has also been studied scientifically. In 2013, the Stanford Research Institute did a study on veterans with PTSD, examining whether weeklong breathing, yoga and meditation workshops helped their symptoms. The study showed that veterans who did the weeklong exercises had decreased PTSD symptoms up to a *year later* compared to the control group, which was a result so positive that it even blew the researchers away—and according to the study, breathwork had the greatest impact.

In the mental health and substance abuse treatment industry, drug addiction and alcohol abuse have been recognized as ways to self-medicate trauma responses. Doing drugs or drinking alcohol are effective at numbing our trauma and unprocessed grief, but once a person becomes physically addicted, they need more and more substances to keep the bad feelings at bay. When they come off those substances, they are even more hyper-sensitive to the feelings they were trying to avoid in the first place. Understanding this is important for anyone getting sober, because simply taking away a coping mechanism for pain doesn't solve the problem. Recovering addicts have to feel their feelings, but almost everyone underestimates how hard that can be after years of avoiding painful emotions with drugs and alcohol. Fortunately, breathwork and meditation can help ease recovering addicts through those difficulties.

Anyone who has gone to AA has likely heard the saying, "let go and let God." It's usually thought of in purely spiritual terms, but it can also be considered in a physical way. All of our heaviest emotions—difficult ones like grief but also uplifting ones like hope and inspiration—are stored and processed in our lungs. Before breathwork, when I heard people say, "let go and let God," I was just confused and annoyed. *Let go of what? I remember thinking. I've already stopped drinking and using, so what else is there to let go of?* After several years of relapses, I finally found out what I needed to let go of: my old ideas on how to live, and my old blocked emotions that were still stuck inside me. I had to surrender my alcohol and drug habits, but I also had to surrender to the feelings I'd been putting off as well.

There's a part in the Big Book of Alcoholics Anonymous that says, "some of us tried to hold on to our old ideas, and the results were nil until we let go absolutely." Though it used to frustrate me, it's now one of my favorite parts—but in order to do what it says, we need to embrace vulnerability and everything that entails. I've discovered that slowing things down and tapping into my parasympathetic nervous system through breathwork helps me let go absolutely. What follows is a deep, still and quiet meditative state, and it's a place where I can do the real work of transformation.

TESTIMONIAL: JOHN'S STORY

For the greater part of my life, I used substances to soothe my pain, both emotional and physical. As I remember, there was a deep void within me, and I felt different from everyone else. I was not worthy or likable, and I didn't feel safe in this world—in fact, the world was a very fearful and unkind place for me.

At the age of five, I experienced what it was like to get drunk for the first time and my entire world changed. As the saying goes, "I had found my solution to my unease." From that point on, I would sneak sips of drinks when adults set them down and grab at others' cocktails whenever I could. My very early start progressed over the years into a major physical, mental and spiritual issue.

Since I had such limited access to alcohol as a child, I reached for sugar instead and started craving it daily. I became obese, and in adolescence and young adulthood, I started abusing alcohol and other substances weekly as soon as I was able to. From my late 20s to late 40s, I used some kind of substance every day, even though it was just a temporary solution for my deeper pathology. The real issues were within myself.

Self-hatred, denial, worthlessness and selfishness penetrated every part of my life and started to affect all my personal relationships and the people I attracted to me. Finally, I had my first awakening in a hospital in 2012, when I was diagnosed with acute pancreatitis as a result of alcohol poisoning and other addictions, and I was given only a 40 percent chance of survival. At that point, my journey to sobriety began, and I knew that it was do or die.

I've been on the path of improvement and healing for 11 years since, always trying to restore the real me that I escaped so early in life. I've made tremendous strides and can confidently say I am not the same man I was 10 years ago. I joined a fellowship, adapted to having spirituality in my life, took an inventory of myself and examined my patterns. I began to treat others with more kindness, honesty and openness, and I grew compassion for myself and others. I became a sober seeker of my true self.

Gradually, I began to dabble in meditation and I concentrated on my breathing to calm myself. I read and listened to spiritual teachers, inspirational speakers and neuroscientists. Over time, I got the feeling that there was another path for me, easier than the one I'd been following—one that I truly believed could lead to a better life. Even so, each morning I still woke up with the feeling of "coming to" in a foxhole.

My fear and anxiety still existed, and I was hyper-alert to my surroundings and feelings of depression and terror, all of which I recognized from childhood and adolescence. Though I was sober from drugs and alcohol, I still reached for any stimulus I could get to soothe my body and mind—whether that was strong coffee, something sweet, a couple of cigarettes or some drama on the news. Every few days, I had to manage my uncomfortable feelings until I got back to fellowship for a renewal of faith and an influx of spirit. I had made progress, but I knew the solution was incomplete.

After a few brief relapses (which I prefer to call "adjustments"), I reached out for help and the universe brought Nick Terry and me together. Nick started to teach me about his approach to breathwork, introducing me to simple skills before moving on to more advanced techniques. We focused on making daily progress in breath practice, and we constantly exchanged hopeful and grateful thoughts. We also shared time reading and learning together about mindful breathing and other spiritual practices through the teachings of people like Eckhart Tolle, all of which helped me come to terms with how I was thinking and feeling, as well as how I was interpreting my life.

Slowly but surely, I became hooked on my breath practice. It took me to a place in mind, body and spirit that I had never been able to reach on my own throughout the years. Finally, things were shifting. I regained the hunger to expand my life, along with a hopefulness that things would be okay. I surrendered to my routine of breathwork, meditation and honest words from the wise people around me. I was open-minded and ready to grow, willing to put in the necessary work for change.

Today, I no longer reach for any other stimulus when I wake up. Each day, I begin with some stretching before sitting for a moment to conjure up good energy and develop a positive relationship with myself. I start with some deep breathing and chanting, then settle into my mantras, deconstructing any labels I still have about myself. After that, I do my prayers and continue with intense breathwork. I use the Wim Hof method in the morning since it brings such substantial benefits, though I use other methods throughout the day to find ease when I need to. Afterwards, I generally sit for a short meditation before beginning my day.

Today, I can modulate my mood and chronic pain through my routine and my breathing techniques. I don't need to use alcohol, drugs, cigarettes, sugar or news to create drama in my *life. All my choices are aimed at feeling, instead of punishing myself.*

In the beginning, I found it quite difficult to get motivated for my routine. I was fearful of the breathwork each morning. "What if I fail?" I thought to myself. "I can't do this; it's such a chore." Even so, I stuck with it. Today, I have almost two years of continuous daily breath practice behind me. Though I sometimes don't feel like it, I push on anyway, and at some point during the exercises, my breathing takes over just like it did at the very beginning. Every time, it reminds me of that feeling when the training wheels came off my bicycle for the first time, and I started to glide without falling down—or when a runner suddenly gets their "second wind" and no longer feels the struggle to keep going. And none of it would have been possible without working with Nick.

Thanks again, Nick, for all you do and for giving me the opportunity to reflect and grow. I am more connected to my truth than I have ever been. Love you, brother. Aloha!

6

CONNECTION (SPIRITUAL, EMOTIONAL, PHYSICAL)

Diseases of addiction and depression tend to put us in a state of darkness, loneliness and isolation. Put another way, they put us in a profound state of disconnection, and the solution for these afflictions is to seek the opposite and find a state of connection. Everyone has heard about the importance of connection, but we don't always understand that it takes many different forms. As simply as possible, there is spiritual connection (with a greater power and the world at large), emotional connection (through honesty with yourself and others about your feelings) and physical connection (through the conditioning of your own body and engaging with the world around you).

By becoming more connected, we can transform and grow personally, interpersonally and spiritually: the three kinds of relationships we can have in this world. Our relationship with ourselves involves our self-image and our sense of self-esteem, both of which we can take the time to develop, while our spiritual relationships are what Eckhart Tolle calls "our relationships with being," encompassing the entire world and our understanding of it. Finally, our interpersonal relationships are what we have with other people. Unfortunately, most people coming into recovery are fairly broken in all three areas, though most universal among addicts is the damaged sense of self-image.

Since most addicts are broken in all forms of connection, a big part of the recovery process is to learn how to create or recreate those relationships. It's important not to skip any of the three, because anything we don't work on or develop will be a place where we get blocked, which can lead to dissatisfaction and frustration, along with the kind of thought spirals that lead to relapse. In my own recovery, I was resistant to change in all three areas at different times, and sometimes simultaneously. In general, the one I worked on the most at first was my relationship with myself.

When I first started going to meetings, I heard people talking about recovery being all about relationships. I wondered, *What the hell do relationships have to do with not drinking and using?* I also thought, *I certainly hope recovery is not about relationships, because I have no clue how to do them.* I didn't realize how much that extended to my relationship with myself as well. A big shift for me came when I met a woman in recovery who said, "You're not who *you* think you are, you're not who *they* think you are, and you're certainly not who *you* think *they* think you are." It was confusing, and led to the question: *Who am I?*

Over time, I was able to run through all kinds of things I *wasn't.* I managed to separate from my thoughts and patterns, observing them to see what was left over. Both breathwork and meditation were invaluable here, and I wish I'd done them earlier as I could've saved myself some time. While there's no single answer to the "who am I" question, the best one I've come up with is that *I am a spiritual being having a human experience.* I am connected to the source, and I am enough. I also believe that no man is an island, and our entire existence is relational to the world around us. It took a long time to untangle that woman's riddle, but this is my best attempt.

In the process of working on my relationship with myself, it was impossible to avoid my relationship with spirituality, since it was the jumping-off point of my 12-Step program. Even so, I was constantly confused by what God was and what it all meant. Initially, I prayed even when I didn't know why I was doing it, and I drew connections between things that seemed too miraculous not to be a little bit divine. It happened when I ran into Sean at the airport on the way to my uncle's wedding, as well as when I worked through my inventory and got a glimpse of what it meant to "let go." Perhaps more than anything else, it all clicked for me through breathwork and meditation: when I saw that while I might be separate from my thoughts, I am not separate from God. As the observer of my thoughts, I was one with God and the universe. That truth was always with me, and I could tap into it every day.

To improve my relationship with myself and my spirituality, I dug deep into my inventory to find the root causes of things, and I sought to forgive myself and others. Doing so allowed me to view myself in a new way. I was able to disconnect from the conditioning of my childhood and my past behaviors, and start over from a place of forgiveness and liberation. My other major resource was my breathwork. Through deep breathing exercises, I stimulated my vagus nerve, the largest in the nervous system, to help regulate my mood and lower inflammation. Since inflammation is at the root of countless mental and physical health issues, lowering mine has helped me stay as present as possible, and to be the best I can be every day. All of this prepared me to look at my relationships with others—particularly my romantic relationships—which was its own major challenge.

After several years of sobriety, I went to my sponsor Phil and explained my relationship struggles in full. Right away, he saw my brokenness, and he told me that I was in no position to be in a romantic relationship with anyone else. For the many years I was in and out of rooms, treatment centers and sober living homes, I was looking at girls almost every chance I got. I was trying to catch someone's eye just like I always had. I was still acting like a 16-year-old boy in an adult's body.

During that period, I always found willing participants to have sex with. After all, that's what I thought a relationship was: sex. A part of me really wanted to find love and true connection in early sobriety, but I wanted to do so by having sex first. I thought physical connection might lead to what I was looking for, but whenever I hooked up with someone, all that followed was emptiness. It was the same story that had followed me my entire life. I was bringing all my broken childhood tools into my adult life. I didn't know how to live with someone else or how to be a good partner, and as a result, I was struggling.

As Phil explained, sex in early recovery is often just drugs in another person's body: until we get ourselves under control, sex can be a temporary fix for a bigger, structural problem. For the first few years of sobriety, I tried my best to walk the path of recovery and live an ethical sexual life. Ultimately, what I learned was that the "no relationships" rule in early recovery wasn't made up to punish anyone. It was a real protection to stop newly-sober people from getting distracted—and from hurting others. By following my sponsor's advice as best as I could, I finally *did* find love in a way that felt complete and whole, and didn't leave me feeling empty. Of course, it took many years of hard work to reach that point.

Through all the recovery work we do in our three big relationships—spiritual, personal and interpersonal—the commonality is that we start to overcome our egocentrism, which is a hallmark of addiction and alcoholism. Egocentrism is the idea that the world revolves around us, and what we want matters more than what anyone else wants. It's a common trait of an adolescent brain, or the brain of anyone who hasn't grown up yet—and as I learned firsthand, I had an adolescent brain until I was about 34 years old.

I was constantly looking at the world from the perspective of what was in it for me, not thinking of others. When I finally moved away from that, I began to consider everything as a whole and how other people felt. I explored what life was about and where I fit into it. From that foundation, I started to genuinely care about people, and became more concerned with helping others than helping myself. All of this transformed my self-image, which helped me move towards spiritual principles of honesty, hope, faith, courage, willingness, integrity, humility, justice, love, perseverance, spirituality and service.

Practicing all these principles regularly has led to a life of connection in every sense of the word. Though I still sometimes slip into my thoughts and feel distant from myself and others, keeping a regular breathwork practice helps me get back on the right path and in touch with who I am. Maintaining connection has enabled me to live free from drugs, alcohol and disruptive behaviors. It's not magic; it's the regular practice of spiritual principles, and I know the same thing is possible for others as well.

7

PERSEVERANCE

Sometimes the only secret of success is not to do anything differently but to *not* do anything differently...and just be patient. I've found this to be true in recovery as well, but it can be a difficult trap to avoid for anyone who isn't aware of it. Since recovery from addiction isn't a magic pill but a lifelong process, it's normal to feel very aligned on some days and less aligned on others. This is also the nature of living a spiritual life, however frustrating that might be.

Living a truly connected life can feel alien to people who have been in active addiction for many years. For people who are out of practice, it can drain their energy very quickly. In a sense, the ability to connect with ourselves and others is a muscle that must be developed. Doing so takes practice, and it also requires perseverance, despite any difficulties or delays on the way to success. As a spiritual principle, perseverance is absolutely indispensable for long-term recovery.

Anyone who has been around the rooms of recovery is probably familiar with the clichés and sayings that can seem a little cheesy and redundant. Telling someone to persevere in the face of adversity sounds like another cliché, even though it's completely true. One saying that I'm particularly fond of comes directly from AA: "You're only as sick as your secrets." It seems easy enough to understand on the surface, but there's a lot of depth to it.

When it comes to getting sober, there's an initial period that feels like a purge, when we catch up on everything we've ever lied about or done wrong. We do our inventory, we start making amends and we help others, and all that change can feel like a high in itself—resulting in what some have called the "pink cloud" of early recovery. But once that initial rush fades away, we still have a lot of our old patterns and we still make a lot of wrong choices; we just pay less attention to them now that we've started doing *some* of the right things. In a sneaky way, we give our ego permission to come in through the back door.

Addiction is a progressive, patient and often deadly disease, and it's worth saying that directly so as not to sugarcoat things. Though it's great to do all the upfront work of getting honest and making amends, it's also important to remember that the kinds of "secrets" that make us sick can be an accumulation of tiny things that build up over time, things we don't notice until it's too late. Throughout any given week, we have dozens or hundreds of interactions with other people and tons of chances to do great things—but we also have countless opportunities to tell white lies, be selfish and deviate from our principles. Over time, and without proper self-reflection and accountability, those little slips can add up, and we can find ourselves right back where we started.

I've witnessed many people not being entirely truthful, keeping secrets and not living a transparent life, and they often end up relapsing on some substance or self-destructive behavior. I take this very seriously, because with almost all the relapses I've had in my life and the ones I've seen over the course of my sobriety, some kind of built-up dishonesty was the cause. In 12-Step recovery, as in most spiritual practices, one of the biggest, most constant demands is that we always be as honest as possible—and that can be incredibly frustrating and demoralizing at times.

One of the tallest hurdles in 12-Step communities is the initial identification structure that they have in place: "Hi, my name is Nick, and I'm a depressed, anxious and compulsive alcoholic, addict, liar, sex fiend, gambler and overall powerless person! And I'm grateful to be here." In a few subtle ways, forcing this kind of speech creates a lot of opportunities for dishonesty and performance. For one thing, maybe we *aren't* grateful but feel obliged to say we are. And sometimes we *don't* feel completely powerless anymore, but we feel like we have to say it to fit into the crowd.

I understand the intention behind these identifiers, but after being sober for seven years and working in the field for six, I've found that most people don't want to be reduced to a list of problems, and rightfully so. While it's important to understand that addiction and mental illness are real and we need to do the right things to keep them at bay, it isn't necessarily useful to turn every single problem we have into a permanent label. In a sense, it's the same concept as differentiating from our thoughts to observe them.

Believing that we *are* our thoughts is one of the biggest mistakes we make as humans. Not being able to stop thinking is probably the most harmful compulsive addiction there is, but we often don't realize it; after all, everybody thinks, so it's considered normal. I got sober in AA and I'm still grateful for the principles, but from the very beginning, I thought the "I'm an alcoholic for the rest of my life" introduction was over the top. I put that concern aside because I was in pain and I badly needed help, but I think about that introduction differently today. I believe that permanently identifying with the image of an addict or alcoholic creates a variety of different concepts, judgments, words, distractions and definitions that can block our purest relationships with body, soul and spirit, even if those labels can be helpful for a while.

Ego-driven identification comes between you and yourself, between you and your fellows, between you and nature and between you and God. Because of this, you need to ask yourself: is the way you identify more harmful or helpful in your journey toward physical, emotional and spiritual sobriety? There's no one answer to this question, but it's one worth contemplating. If the AA introduction bothers you but the rest of the 12 Steps resonate, I'm here to give you permission to identify however you want in this present moment. Being an "addict" or "alcoholic" is not necessarily the core essence of who we are. As I think of them today, they are patterns of thought cycles that can flare up again and again, and each time, we have to release them.

When old emotional pain bodies arise or trauma response patterns flare up in my life, I pause, take a deep breath in and hold my breath before letting it go slowly. I repeat this pattern whenever I'm irritated, fearful, worried or doubtful. By taking a deep breath in and pausing before responding or reacting, I save myself from discord and chaos—and I find that whatever "I" am still remains after the feelings pass.

If for some reason I do react in a manner that's inconsistent with my new values, I try to take ownership and admit my wrongs. I must be quick to see my part in problems and even quicker to disregard others' faults. This entire recovery life is about looking inward, because my own reactions are the only ones I truly have power over. This is not an overnight lesson; for me, I know it will take continuous practice for the rest of my life. Whenever dishonesty, resentment, fear, jealousy and shame re-emerge, I take a deep breath in and ask the spirit to take them away and bring me back to the present—then I let those emotions go. If the feelings keep returning in a way I can't control by doing the right things and breathing, then I always discuss them with someone else. (Don't keep secrets!)

The tricky thing about perseverance is that even the name sets us up to fail. It plays into another major trap that so many of us fall into, which is the trap of time. In reality, time is an illusion—and yet humans spend their lives counting every second in every minute of every day, week, month, year, decade and century. The only real thing that exists, the only place and time we can be sober, is in the present. If we think about it that way, then "perseverance" doesn't really exist, since it implies time. Our goal should always be to do the right thing, right now. If abstinence is the goal, which for me it absolutely is, then sobriety from this moment to the next should be the longest period of time that we focus on.

The biggest challenge I've seen for people who struggle to put together extended periods of sobriety is the inherent shame that comes with relapse, and having to reintroduce themselves as newcomers. I was "new" in 12-Step meetings for six years when I couldn't maintain abstinence for longer than 60 days. The point is that if you've put together some time and picked up a drink or a drug, or engaged in a behavior you promised to stop, it's okay. Beating yourself up over it or getting overly attached to the idea of either long-term sobriety or a short-term relapse won't do you any good. All that will help you is staying sober this moment, and into the next.

While time isn't real, our feelings of guilt, shame, regret and remorse *are* real in the moment, and we can heal them by being vulnerable enough to feel them and persevere through them. By doing that, we can stop focusing on counting time and come back to our center. The ego always wants to attach itself to the past or the future, and it can only do so with the construct of time. Don't let it. In those moments, continue to breathe, look inward and admit the places where you might be stubborn or wrong. Don't worry about what other people think or say, just come back. Come back home.

8

SERVICE AND SPIRITUAL CURRENCY

Service to acquire spiritual currency isn't really a principle in itself; instead, it's a relationship that emerges by doing *everything* before it, and making all the previous steps a part of your life.

By adopting those practices, positive things beyond our control start to happen, and we pay more attention to the mystery in the connections between things.

We develop a sense of wonder and awe about life instead of a sense of despair and hopelessness. At its core, this is what true spirituality looks like—and it's important to remember that it isn't something we can cling to or possess. It's something we must continually cultivate, and one of the best ways to do so is to encourage similar awakenings in other people. One of the most helpful concepts for me as it relates here is the idea of "spiritual currency."

Spiritual currency is what I call living wholeheartedly and being centered in service to others. It's the abundance of wealth that flows through us when we're connected to a higher purpose or an inner calling toward creative altruism and service. The freedom and meaning I've found from doing this have been like hitting the spiritual lottery—but the only catch is that in order to keep any of it, you have to give it all away. All of it. The more you give away, the more you acquire—and the more you acquire, the more you have to give. If you can do that, the pipeline of abundance can be never-ending.

In my life, my service to others started by giving people rides to meetings and other recovery gatherings. It started with making coffee for others in AA, and then being a secretary, a treasurer and serving on committees that taught me lifelong lessons about selflessness and altruism. As it turns out, Alcoholics Anonymous was founded on this kind of spiritual altruism. When Bill Wilson couldn't free himself from the grasp of alcohol, he was approached by Ebi Thatcher, a friend who'd gotten sober with religion. Ebi offered to help Bill if he was willing. Even though Bill wasn't religious, his friend told him he could choose whatever concept of God he wanted—and that was when a shift occurred. Bill had never considered that he could have his own idea of God, free from religious dogma and stigma—and as a result, he had his first internal spiritual experience.

Bill ended up hospitalized for the last time after that meeting with Ebi, and he had another spiritual experience in the hospital. He realized that at his core, he was connected to a real spiritual force, one that exists behind everything in the universe. This overwhelming feeling was followed by the certainty that he'd only be able to stay sober if he carried this message to other struggling alcoholics. So that's what he did.

This altruistic impulse brought Bill to hospitals and psych wards, where he shared his message of hope with other alcoholics—but after six months, he was the only one still sober. None of the people he tried to help stopped drinking, even though his ideas had worked for him, and he felt filled with purpose for the first time in his life. Sometime later, Bill found himself in a hotel lobby in Akron, Ohio, upset after a recent business venture had gone sideways. He was feeling stressed because money was tight, and depression and self-pity were setting in. He could see the bar across the lobby where drinks were clinking and jazz music was playing. He immediately went to the phone booth and started calling numbers, trying to find a suffering alcoholic to talk to.

Finally, Bill started calling churches, asking if anybody knew an alcoholic in need of help. He was given the phone number of Dr. Bob Smith, an Akron physician who'd been losing his battle with alcoholism for several years. Bill got in touch with Bob's wife, and she invited him over. When Bill arrived at Dr. Bob's house, his wife showed him where Bob was lying down.

"You've got 10 minutes, mister," proclaimed Dr. Bob, "and I don't want your help."

"Good," Bill said. "I'm not here to help you. I'm here to help myself. I don't want to drink again, and if I don't help another alcoholic, I'm sure to drink again, and if I drink again, I'll die." The two men sat and talked for hours—and that's how AA started.

Years later, both men died sober, never having had another drink. They carried their message of creative altruism and hope to the first one hundred recovered people in AA, and one hundred turned into one hundred thousand. Today, there's four hundred 12-Step programs and millions of recovered members all over the world.

The point of me telling this now-infamous story isn't to plug AA, though I do admire and respect the program. Instead, it's to illustrate how powerful it is for one person to try to help another overcome their problems. Over the years, I've worked with hundreds of men who have suffered as tremendously as I did with drug and alcohol addiction, mental health and compulsion. Every one of them, without exception, had extremely low self-esteem, which often led to drowning in shame and self-pity. The cure for that shame is always excruciating vulnerability and courageous service to others. Dr. Martin Luther King Jr. once said, "Life's most urgent and persistent question is, 'What are you doing for others?'" To this day, it's a question I ask myself all the time.

The illusion of separateness is what keeps us locked in the pain of selfishness, self-delusion, self-pity and self-righteousness. It often keeps us living in two fantasy realms: the past or the future. Breathwork and meditation, on the other hand, connect us to the present moment where everything exists—breath, love, spirit and God. While there's no one way to tap into the present moment and realize how connected we all are, my prescription for a more conscious and enlightened experience is simple: in the morning, do a full body scan for awareness, say a quick prayer, and then begin a breathwork routine. As you practice your routine, you can increase your reps and the length of your breath holds, but remember that time isn't the goal. The goal is to go into your body, connect with spirit and soul, and change your nervous system to allow that to be possible.

After doing this, I also recommend grabbing a pen and paper and writing down three things you're grateful for and three things that will help make that day a good one. Next, write down a list of "I am" affirmations that help you visualize your truest, most authentic purpose. For example:

I am an amazing author.
I am an incredible artist.
I am unconditionally loved.
I am connected to source.
I am source.

Throughout the day, whenever you get frustrated, insecure, angry, uncertain or doubtful, take a moment to breathe deeply through your nose for a few seconds, hold your breath at the top for several seconds, then slowly exhale. When you first begin, count for four seconds as you breathe in deep through the nose. After that, hold for seven seconds and exhale for eight. Keep this pattern in your pocket and use it as often as you'd like throughout the day. Use if before a challenging situation, during and after.

Make a habit of scanning your consciousness and asking yourself: *Is there anything I need to share with someone? A mentor, sponsor, respected friend or coach? Am I keeping secrets? Am I being honest with myself? Am I fearful? Am I harboring any resentments?* If you can rest with a clear conscience, then all is well; if you need to talk with someone, plan accordingly. This is the spiritual solution. It's the awakening of your spirit in the present moment, also known as the fourth dimension of existence. This is all there's ever been and all there will ever be.

One of the biggest takeaways I've learned through recovery is that nothing is more helpful than having a passion for doing kind things for others without any expectation in return. I learned it through community, spirituality and a relationship with a higher power of the universe—whether it's Ke'Akua, Allah, Buddha or Jesus. To this day, I maintain a sense of spirituality by searching inwardly through prayer, breathwork and meditation, and by serving others whenever I can.

Practicing prayer, breathwork and meditation nourishes and feeds the soul in the same way sunshine, water and healthy food nourishes and feeds the body. There is a direct connection between self-reflection, prayer, breathwork, cold water exposure and meditation. When practiced separately, any one of these can be beneficial—but when braided together, they create an inseparable union of spirit, breath and soul.

TESTIMONIAL: TRAVIS'S STORY

I've struggled with anxiety and addiction my entire adult life, and I encountered breathwork at one point while I was still using. At the time, I paid little attention to it; I didn't know all the benefits it could offer for people in recovery. Things didn't really change for me until I found myself in treatment again, where I met Nick Terry.

Nick and I connected immediately through our common interest in surfing and other outdoor activities in Hawaii. He explained his approach to breathwork and all the benefits it could offer, especially for people who had tried to get sober in other ways and couldn't make it stick. After explaining to me how it all worked, Nick got me started on a regular breathwork routine in addition to all the other things I was doing for my recovery.

The anxiety I experienced in the first few weeks of sobriety was nearly unbearable. There were plenty of moments when my hands would get clammy, my body would tense up and my heart would race. Just like Nick promised, the only thing that gave me real relief from those symptoms was breathwork—whenever I dropped into the exercises, my hands would dry, my body would relax and I could finally calm down. Nick helped me so much in learning that there were other ways of breathing, thinking and being. It was an incredible gift, and from that moment on, I knew I would carry it with me forever.

For anyone struggling with depression, anxiety or substance abuse, or who simply wants to elevate their life, take it from Nick: breathwork is the answer. Just like anything else though, it's not a one-and-done kind of thing. However powerful it is, you will still have to apply yourself. You'll have to dig deep when you do it, especially on days when you don't want to.

Spiritually and emotionally, breathwork and meditation have given me more than any substance or medication ever could (or ever will). It's something I would wish for everyone looking for recovery, and I have Nick Terry to thank for it.

CONCLUSION

Of all the important and transformational things I've learned on my long journey to recovery is this: by surrendering the old ways, letting go and letting God, life in sobriety is more exciting and full than it ever was before. Aside from doing all the "right" things and improving life for yourself and your loved ones, it's also true that recovery is just plain fun—and opening yourself up to life and to the idea of spiritual currency can take you places you never thought possible. Just to illustrate, I want to share one last story.

About six months after I opened my treatment center, Honu House Hawaii, I started working with my cousin to help him heal his anxiety and panic attacks with a breathwork routine. He had recently completed a treatment program in Utah after many attempts to get sober on his own, and we decided to go on an expedition in Spain together: a 120-person retreat in the Pyrenees mountains with one of my all-time heroes, Wim Hof. Out of all the people with whom I've shared breathwork and cold water exposure, my cousin is the only one who's become a true convert. Though I'd never met Wim Hof before, I first learned about breathwork by watching his videos online and by that point, I'd modeled much of my life after his teachings. I couldn't wait for the trip.

When the day finally came, Wim and his instructors demonstrated his methods, including how long to breathe, what made the process work and what the results of it would be. As they explained, for new people, the standard exercise was one to two minutes of breathwork and cold exposure in one of three big ice pools his team had prepared. After the introduction, Wim took over.

"Alright," he yelled in his signature accent. "We're going 10 minutes in the ice, everybody in!" Almost immediately, everyone panicked—including his instructors, who had just explained that the cold plunges would only be one to two minutes. In response to the crowd's general malaise and confusion, Wim kept shouting cheerfully and leading the way by taking his clothes off and getting in one of the ice baths. "Just follow me," he hollered. "Remember, we are the alchemists, and we're going for 10 minutes!"

Even if many of the people in the crowd were uncertain, everyone gradually jumped in. Since I'd been doing daily breathwork and cold exposure back in Hawaii, the 10 minutes didn't seem like it would be a problem. Sure enough, doing the Wim Hof method together in a group *with* Wim Hof added some extra encouragement and motivation, and nearly everyone made it the full 10 minutes before we all jumped out again. With the cold plunge behind us, everyone was relaxed and in a great mood. Wim pulled out a drum and everyone formed a circle around him as he started talking about all kinds of things, from Big Pharma to organic food. About 20 minutes later, Wim abruptly put the drum down and stood up.

"I'm going back in the ice!" he shouted, jumping back into one of the pools. This time, the crowd was much less eager to follow him. *This is my chance*, I thought. Before I could think about it too much, I stripped down again and approached him.

"May I join you?" I asked, and he waved me in warmly.

"Yes, come in!" he boomed. With that, I climbed back in and started telling him my story: how I'd gotten sober and opened my own treatment center, about all the people I had worked with and how much his teachings had helped me.

Wim lit up. "Amazing!" he said. "I think of unprocessed trauma in the same way with the ice and the breath—with the breath, we are lifting it out. We are the alchemists!" We had been talking so long that 10 minutes had passed and I was starting to really feel the cold, but I kept breathing deeply and nodded.

"That's been a huge motivation for me," I told him. "We have clinical therapists, doctors, and high-level, evidence-based practices at our center, and people tell me privately that the breath work is the most important practice they learned. The breath isn't a replacement for therapy, but it's a tool to create the space where true healing can begin."

After I told him this, Wim beamed. "We have to do an interview!" With that, he gestured to one of his cameramen to come and record us. After one of the camera assistants counted us in and called action, Wim started introducing himself and explaining the situation.

"And here we are with Nick," he said, "on his *second time in the ice!* Nick, say it again, what you just told me!" As the rest of the guests gathered around to watch our interview, I explained more about my life in Hawaii, the work we do at the recovery center and how I believe breathwork is an integral missing piece to the mental health and substance abuse puzzle. Finally, after much longer than recommended in the ice bath, we got out and toweled off.

The next day, after the usual exercises, there was a big

Q&A session with Wim, and everyone asked him questions about his breathing techniques. Eventually, one PhD-level therapist stood at the microphone to ask him a question.

"Your work is so awesome," the therapist said. "How do I get this message out to all the people who need it most?" Hearing this, Wim started scanning the room.

"Where's the guy from Hawaii?" he shouted. My heart started racing as I slowly held up my hand. "Get up here; tell him what you said to me!" As I started walking toward the stage, so many thoughts were running through my head. *I was expelled from high school and only finally finished my degree at 35*, I thought. *Now, Wim Hof is asking me to explain to a PhD-level therapist how to bring breathwork to his clients.*

"Well, this is a lot more qualitative than quantitative," I began, "but here's what I've noticed." Once again, I described the work I'd done at my treatment center in Hawaii, trying to keep my composure the whole time. "Breathwork isn't a *replacement* for trauma therapy," I said, "but it is something that can access it. You can 'feel it to heal it', which helps you work through it. What I've found is that it can help people face trauma and discard it rather than circulating it forever." Finally, I gave the microphone back and the crowd burst into applause.

For the rest of the retreat, our group kept doing breathing exercises and ice baths, all while hiking through the mountains and exploring the rugged landscape. On the last day, all 120 of us went on a beautiful hike up into the Pyrenees mountains surrounded by magnificent waterfalls. At the top of the mountain range there was a photo opportunity for all of the attendees to get a picture or selfie with Wim Hof himself with the most magical backdrop. A few days early I had performed some spoken word/rap lyrics during a talent contest that everyone seemed to love, especially Wim. When it was my turn to take a photo with Wim he started to make a beat with his mouth and body, it was incredible, was this really happening?

The lady that was taking the photo signaled to me to start rapping, gesturing that she is now recording with my iPhone. And that was it, I started to rap over Wim Hof's beatbox and everyone was watching. I had a song I had written prior about breathwork and cold water exposure and it just landed perfectly. We ended our organic freestyle rap beat-boxing session with some applause from the crowd and a beautiful embrace with a forehead touch and inhale exhale exchanged. I know it sounds too good to be true. Fortunately I have the video footage to prove all of this on my Instagram account.

On my journey towards surrender, my life got very dark. I was plagued with self-pity, shame, depression, self-centered fear and self-destructive compulsions. Now that I've overcome those deficiencies, my darkest times have become my greatest assets, because I'm uniquely qualified to help others find a light out of the darkness. My journey of creative altruism brought me to where I am right now: writing this book about why breathwork is the missing piece of the spiritual recovery puzzle.

I don't want this book to push any specific dogma or to claim to be the final word on this subject. It's simply about adopting a spiritual way of life in collaboration with a daily breath practice. It's about asking a few simple questions as a way to live a better life: How am I being helpful to others? How can I lift up my fellows? How can I be of service?

These are the questions that will set us free and allow spiritual currency to flow through us and into the people around us. Through all the ups and downs of life, I want people to remind one another the simple truth about the power of our breath.

The very first thing we do when we're born is to take a deep breath in, and the last thing we'll do in the physical realm is exhale before we transition to the other side. In between those two breaths, we can take as many other breaths as we want to, always remembering that it is the breath that carries our soul.

I hope this book has been helpful to you, and if you're ever out our way, I hope to see you at one of Breath of Life Recovery's workshops or support meetings in the future. Until then, *a hui hou mālama pono.*

–Nick Terry, 2023

PART 4

BREATHWORK APPENDIX

INTRODUCTION

To help you on your recovery journey, I've compiled a helpful list of breathwork techniques and exercises here that you can use for various purposes. Keep in mind that you don't have to use all of them; just choose the ones that best fit your needs. If you're feeling down or low, you may gravitate towards the stimulating and activating exercises; on the other hand, if you're anxious and have too much energy, you can try some of the relaxing ones. All of these exercises can be used in conjunction with one another, just do so responsibly and according to their descriptions.

Throughout history, people have used breathwork for so many different purposes, including:

- aiding positive self-development
- boosting immunity
- processing emotions and healing emotional pain
- developing life skills
- developing or increasing self-awareness
- enriching creativity

- improving personal and professional relationships
- increasing confidence, self-image and self-esteem
- increasing joy and happiness
- overcoming addiction
- reducing stress and anxiety
- releasing negative thoughts

Breathwork can be used alongside other interventions to help with all kinds of mental, physical and emotional issues including anger, anxiety, chronic pain, depression, grief, trauma and PTSD. If there's anything I've learned through recovery, it's that the challenges of addiction, alcoholism, depression, grief and trauma are the only prisons for which we already hold the keys. The doors we need to unlock are inside of us, and the breath is the key to unlocking them.

Safety Note: *Some of these exercises can lead to intense experiences at first, including big swells of emotion or anxiety. In some cases (approximately 20 percent in my experience), some people may experience some symptoms of tendonitis after doing breathwork exercises, resulting in tightness in the hands and stiffness. If concerned, you can consult with a doctor, though this is a normal experience that tends to disappear after relaxing.*

Breathwork exercises can be similar to difficult psychedelic experiences, though in a much milder form. In ayahuasca ceremonies or after taking DMT, people commonly feel a "purge" before experiencing benefits; generally speaking, the stronger a person's ego is (their attachment to their identity), the harder the purge will be. Since breathwork can result in changes in perception that feel like a loss of control, these exercises may make you feel tight or tense. When those feelings come up, the best way to proceed is to "feel it to heal it." By not resisting those difficult feelings and allowing them to emerge while knowing they can't hurt you, you can process them and move forward. If we truly believe that trauma and PTSD are at the root of many mental illnesses and addictions, talk therapy may not be sufficient to fully heal them. Instead of burying them, we have to bring these dormant emotions up and out. If you're feeling unsure, stick to exercises that are less intense as you get used to doing breathwork.

BREATH AWARENESS

Before doing breathwork, it's good to start with a breath awareness exercise. It's simple to do, and can help identify what is going on in your body before doing anything else.

1. First, close your eyes and breathe deeply and calmly, focusing on where you hear your breath in your body. Do a slow, full body scan from head to toe to find any tension and hidden feelings. Imagine sending your breath into each area of your body to find these sensations.
2. After breathing for about a minute, pay attention to where your body is moving or twitching as you breathe to understand where you may be holding tension. If possible, ask your body why it feels tension in those places as you continue to slowly breathe.
3. After taking another 30 second pause, shift your focus to feeling your breath as it enters and exits your nostrils. Gradually train your focus so the only

thing in your thoughts is your breath going in
and out.
4. After another 30 seconds to a minute of breathing
    this way, open your eyes. Take note of how you feel
    in your body compared to where you started. What
    differences do you feel physically? What
    differences do you feel emotionally?

This exercise helps to orient ourselves to how the breath moves
through our body, and to establish a mind-body-breath connection that can help us during other exercises. This breath awareness can also be used to alleviate minor feelings of stress or
anxiety, or to refocus on something when we're distracted.

CYCLIC SIGHING
(DOUBLE INHALE BREATHING)

Cyclic Sighing or Double Inhaling is a great breathwork technique that is easy enough for anyone to access, at any level. It taps into the body's natural stress-relieving systems, promoting a sense of calm and lowering anxiety. It can be used to calm down in times of distress, in the evening to get ready for sleep, or in any other context when slowing down and lowering your energy is appropriate.

The technique was recently popularized by Andrew Huberman, a Stanford University neuroscientist, though as he noted the technique is not necessarily one that anyone "invented." Instead, it taps into a reflex called the "physiological sigh," something humans do automatically to regulate stress and clear carbon dioxide from the body.

1. To begin, get in a comfortable seated position with good, upright posture.
2. When you're ready, inhale deeply and relatively quickly through the nose for about two seconds, filling up your lungs.

3. Instead of exhaling, pause very briefly before taking a second quick inhale through the nose for one last "burst" of air; do this for roughly a one-count (or slightly less).
4. After the second inhale, do a long, slow and "sighing" exhale through the mouth for a rough count of four to six (listen to your body here and do what feels comfortable).
5. It is often only necessary to do this technique a few times in a row to significantly lower the stress you feel in your body. As a more structured practice (or in times of greater distress), you can repeat the technique for up to five minutes before stopping and returning your breathing to normal.

Though it may not be best to do this exercise first thing in the morning (as it may make you feel tired), it can be used at any time of day and is very safe and not strenuous when done correctly. While it does involve deep breathing, remember that the purpose is not to energize, push or add stress to the body. The purpose is to *release* stress, which should be kept in mind if you repeat the technique for several minutes rather than doing it only a few times.

After a longer session, your lungs and body may feel somewhat "stretched out," but the feeling should be one of pleasant relaxation, not of strain or tension. If the pace described above causes you to feel pressured or lightheaded, slow each step of the process down in a way that works for you and your body to achieve the desired effects.

4-7-8 BREATHING

For anyone dealing with anxiety and panic, 4-7-8 breathing is an easy, helpful tool to regulate the nervous system that can be done throughout the day:

1. Sit up with your back straight. Exhale completely, forcefully enough to make a whooshing sound.
2. Keeping your mouth closed, put the tip of your tongue on the ridge behind your upper front teeth. Slowly and quietly inhale through the nose while counting to four.
3. Hold your breath while counting to seven.
4. On seven, exhale through your mouth, making another whooshing sound while counting to eight. At eight, your lungs should be empty.
5. Repeat this process three more times, for a total of four cycles.

While this exercise can be good to calm down before going to sleep, it can also be useful before going into a situation that could cause anxiety, such as an important meeting or getting on an airplane. It is useful throughout the day, and as a preventative measure against anxiety and tension. Generally speaking, the technique works by activating the parasympathetic nervous system and shifting the body out of a fight, flight or freeze state.

BOX BREATHING
(SQUARE BREATHING)

Box breathing, or square breathing, is an easy, well-known and often-used technique that can be done at any time of day. It is often used by therapists for clients who have anxiety, and it has been popularized by the Navy SEALs. Box breathing can help relieve tension and bring a person back to a centered state:

1. Sit or lie in a comfortable position with one hand on your chest and one on your stomach. Breathe normally for a minute, taking notice of the rise and fall of your stomach and chest. If your chest is rising but your stomach isn't, this means you're shallow breathing; try to correct this by bringing the breath into the stomach.
2. When you're ready, breathe in slowly through the nose for a count of four seconds.
3. Hold that breath for a count of four seconds.
4. Slowly exhale through your mouth for a count of four seconds.

5. Repeat this process as many times as you need to until you feel centered and relaxed.

As a relaxation technique, box breathing is not stressful on the body and is unlikely to create any intense emotions. Its main uses are to help you refocus if you're distracted or overly energized, to release panic or worry, to correct hyperventilation and restore a normal breathing pattern, and for those with insomnia, to help ease the body into sleep. If the four-second count is too long, the exercise can also be adapted to three seconds.

THREE-PART RESPIRATORY BREATHING

To soften the breathing, activate all parts of the lungs, bring the breath deeper into the body or prepare for meditation, three-part respiratory breathing can be a helpful exercise. As the name suggests, it is one full exercise done in three parts:

1. Begin by sitting on your knees and placing both hands on your belly. Exhale all oxygen through the mouth and then breathe slowly and deeply into the belly as if inflating a balloon, exhaling each time through the mouth.
2. Repeat this process 10 times. On the last inhale, hold for three seconds, place your hands on your knees and then exhale through the mouth. Breathe softly for a few breaths to return to a normal rhythm.
3. In the same position, put both hands on either side of your ribcage and exhale completely through the mouth.

4. Inhale slowly and deeply into the heart center and chest, with the goal of lifting the ribs and floating them upward (doing this may mean hearing a different sound in the nose and chest while breathing than you did in Part I). Exhale through the mouth.

5. Repeat this process 10 times, holding your breath for three seconds on the last inhale. Again, place your palms face up on your knees and release. Breathe slowly and softly for a few moments.

6. Interlock your fingers and put your hands behind your neck, lifting your elbows toward the sky. Exhale completely through the mouth.

7. Inhale slowly and deeply through the nose, focusing on filling the upper part of your lungs and exhaling through the mouth afterwards.

8. Repeat this process 10 times and hold on the last inhale for three seconds while reaching your arms up to the sky.

9. Slowly exhale and place your hands palms up on your knees. Relax and breathe softly and slowly, returning your breath to a normal rhythm.

10. The goal of this exercise is to make your breathing softer and fuller, and to inflate all parts of your lungs. Make your body softer and slower with each repetition, deepening your breath into your body and learning to control your mind. After the exercise is over, you can also go directly into a three-to-five-minute meditation.

11. There are many benefits to this exercise, including gaining control over your respiratory system, oxygenating your body and preparing for meditation. Additionally, the exercise has been

shown to help treating depression and insomnia, as well as asthma, skin problems and various stress disorders.

12. Generally speaking, the lower belly area is known as the "junk drawer" for your emotions, and this exercise is helpful in bringing those emotions up and out of the body. It is also beneficial for good sleep hygiene or sleep dysfunction, as it is a calming exercise that can induce yawning and sleepiness.

STIMULATING BREATH
(I.E. BHASTRIKA OR BELLOWS BREATH)

Originating from Yogic practices as *bhastrika pranayama*, the stimulating or bellows breath is one of the oldest breathing techniques in the world. Originally it was used as a cleansing or preparatory part of a yoga practice. Though it is still useful to add to a yoga practice, it has also been popularized by pro surfer Laird Hamilton, and it can be used on its own to clear the nasal passages and energize the body:

1. Sit up with your spine straight and shoulders relaxed. Bend your elbows and make fists, bringing them up to your shoulders with knuckles facing out and forearms near the torso. Take a normal breath or two in this position before starting.
2. Inhale normally through the nostrils, shooting your arms straight up in the air, opening your hands and spreading your fingers wide. Exhale through the nose with as much force as possible, bringing your arms and fists back to their original position as you do so. This entire process of one breath should take

at most one second. When done correctly, it will sound like hyperventilating.

3. Repeat this process to do 60 breaths within a minute before letting out a long gentle exhale and relaxing the body. This entire routine can be repeated up to three times, with a break of one to two minutes of normal breathing between each one. The repeated cycles can also be done more slowly.

The main purpose of Bhastrika is to increase energy and alertness, so is particularly good for people who feel lethargic. It can also be helpful for people with illnesses that negatively affect their breathing, such as allergies or short-term health issues like bronchitis or the flu. Since this exercise will activate your fight, flight or freeze response, it's also good to use before going to the gym.

In general, the benefits of stimulating breath are that it oxygenates the brain, energizes the nervous system, strengthens immunity and can help ease symptoms of depression and anxiety over time. This exercise is particularly stimulating and can be challenging for those who aren't used to breathing aggressively through the nose. Listen to your body while doing it, and if you feel overly lightheaded, slow the exercise down or do fewer repetitions.

TUMMO BREATHING
(WIM HOF METHOD)

The Wim Hof method is perhaps the most well-known and widely practiced breathwork technique in the Western world, and can be used for many different purposes. Though based on Tibetan Tummo breathing, it has been slightly adapted from its original context and is often used in conjunction with cold plunges or cold exposure.

1. To begin, get into a comfortable position either sitting up straight or lying down.
2. When ready, breathe in deeply and swiftly through the nose, rolling your breath deep from your belly and into your chest like a wave. Once full, exhale swiftly through the mouth until empty and begin inhaling again.
3. Repeat this pattern 30 to 40 times, taking an exaggerated inhale on the last rep before exhaling it all through the mouth.
4. With lungs empty, hold your breath for 30 seconds to a minute, depending on your comfort level.

5. When the time is up, do another deep inhale through the nose and hold for 15 seconds.
6. Relax your body and breathe normally for a moment, before repeating the entire process for a total of two to three rounds.

The Wim Hof breathing method is a stimulating and energizing exercise that is great to do early in the morning, though it's also fine to do throughout the day. Its main benefits are to energize and cleanse your nervous system at a cellular level, as well as oxygenating the body, grounding the mind, boosting the immune system, lowering blood pressure, expanding lung capacity and bringing the mind and body into the present moment.

It is a particularly good tool for addicts and people with mental illness, as it clears the mind of mental chatter, limiting beliefs and other negative self-talk. When done in the morning, it can be a helpful exercise to reset the "narrative" that we tend to begin the day with, replacing it with a blank, positive sense of presence.

UJJAYI BREATHING
(OCEAN BREATHING)

Another technique originating from pranayama and Yogic practices, the Ujjayi breath (or ocean breathing technique) can be used for calming the mind, as well as for cleansing and warming the body. It is mildly stimulating, and can be done at various times throughout the day (though ideally not before bed):

1. Sit up with your back straight and shoulders relaxed, becoming aware of your resting breath pattern. Keep your mouth closed and breathe normally through your nose only.
2. Bring your awareness to your throat, and begin to slightly tighten it to restrict the air coming in. You can also imagine breathing "through" the throat, or breathing from higher up in the neck than you usually would. When done correctly, the inhale will sound like a soft hissing or scraping sound: this is the air passing through the tightened opening of your throat.

3. After enough air has entered your lungs this way, begin to exhale slowly, again hearing that same hissing sound. This textured in-out sound is why it is also called ocean breathing, as it mimics the sounds of waves crashing in and out on the shore.

The benefits of this exercise are that it warms up the internal organs, which helps to cleanse them, and that it gently raises your energy levels, improves concentration and releases tension. This is a good exercise to use for a boost, either before work or before exercise. For those who practice yoga, this breathing technique can be used throughout the duration of a yoga session, as it helps to control the breath and mind while making stretching easier.

As a safety precaution, anyone with asthma should be cautious when doing this exercise. Be sure you are still getting enough air and don't continue if you feel lightheaded or nauseous. Remember to constrict the throat only slightly to still allow enough air to flow through. To ease into this exercise, it can also be done with the mouth slightly open to make sure enough air enters the lungs.

ALTERNATE NOSTRIL BREATHING

This technique is one of many that originates from Yogic practices of pranayama, sometimes also called shamanic breathwork techniques. Alternate nostril breathing can be used on its own or as a part of rebirthing breathwork, which combines it with other circular breathing techniques to regulate the emotions.

1. Begin by sitting up in a comfortable position with your spine straight. Put your right hand on your belly and the other hand on your forehead.
2. Using your left thumb, cover your right nostril and inhale deeply through the left nostril.
3. When your lungs are full, lift your thumb and use your pointer finger to cover your left nostril and exhale through your right nostril. When these steps are done correctly, you will inhale through the left nostril and exhale through the right nostril for each breath, with your left hand alternately pinching off each side between breaths.

4. Repeat this process for two to 10 minutes, remembering to keep your breathing as smooth and continuous as possible throughout. When you're done, let your body relax and your breathing return to normal.

This exercise can be very helpful in opening up the nasal passages and preparing you for other breathwork techniques. As a gentle and relaxing technique, it has the benefits of lowering anxiety, lowering blood pressure, regulating the nervous system and calming the mind. For these and other reasons, it can also be used as preparation for yoga or meditation.

CLARITY BREATHING AND BREATH OF LIFE

Another longer breathwork exercise, clarity breathing, or Breath of Life, is an intensive way to process blockages, stresses and emotions in the body.

1. Begin by lying down on your back somewhere you won't be disturbed. Place your hands on your lower belly and feel yourself breathing normally for a few moments.
2. When you're ready to begin, do a two-part inhale, starting by filling up the belly and then rolling the breath into the chest like a wave.
3. Once your lungs are full, exhale hard and fast through the mouth. When done correctly, this should make a loud but whispered *ha* sound.
4. Repeat this process without pausing for anywhere between five to 45 minutes depending on your comfort level and experience. As you complete the session, focus on moving your breath all throughout your body and using it to find "blockages." As you

find each blockage, keep breathing until you've released the blockage and continue scanning.

5. When the exercise is over, relax and allow your breathing to return to normal. For anyone with a yoga practice, you can also transition directly into Child's Pose to ease back into your day.

The benefits of transformational breathing include improved function of the entire respiratory system, greater oxygenation of the body, improved circulation, organ detoxification, improved energy levels, stress relief and improved trauma symptoms. More generally, the practice can result in long-term, positive changes to the autonomic nervous system, improved mental and emotional states, more balanced and even energy levels and a greater sense of spiritual connection.

As with other long and intense breathwork techniques, beginners shouldn't do transformational breathing without supervision! Though this exercise can be longer or shorter depending on the person's comfort level, it is designed to initially stimulate the body's fight, flight or freeze response before gradually moving through that response. As such, it may bring up difficult emotions and experiences, and may not be suitable for people with epilepsy, high blood pressure, cardiovascular disease, neurological issues or who are pregnant or breastfeeding.

WORK WITH NICK TERRY TNT

WWW.BREATHOFLIFERECOVERY.ORG

After two heart failures and a crazy pandemic, I recognized that I needed to try a new path for my health. I had the opportunity and good fortune to spend two months on Maui with Nick Terry building my strength with much needed breathwork and meditation. Nick was extraordinarily helpful, both by giving me daily "workouts" and educating me about his processes. I now have a regimen I have been able to implement back home in New York City to fulfill the promise of our work. I cannot speak highly enough of the gentleman and our experience together.

—Andrew Martin-Weber, Broadway Producer

Aloha! My experience at The Recovery Center with Nick Terry has had remarkable benefits in my life, particularly through the daily practice of breathwork. In his classes, Nick introduced me to many different forms, styles and techniques of breathing that have allowed my body to take control over my thoughts. By improving my focus, mental outlook and clarity, these techniques have continued to have a profound influence on me every day, and my meditation practice has become easier, deeper and more beneficial. Please take advantage of Nick and his teachings; they are an opportunity to change your life for the better.

—Tom Barry, Retired General Contractor

Initially, I was skeptical about breathwork. I've been suffering from anxiety, depression, self-harm and insomnia my entire life. How can breathing, which is something I do all day, every day, actually make a difference? It's amazing how wrong I was. After even just one session of breathwork with Nick Terry, I began to feel like I had an outlet for my panicked mind. Though the first time was under the perfect setting of a cotton candy sunrise before surfing, I've found that as I continue to progress, I'm able to stabilize myself through breathwork even in un-ideal settings and circumstances.

Many of us suffer from not being able to live in the present or take a step back from ourselves to relieve anxiety. Breathwork with Nick has reduced my anxiety and insomnia all together. I finally feel mindful and at peace in my own body, and the fact that it's something I can do at any time without needing anything but air is remarkable. I am so grateful for Nick. His energy and aura when teaching breathwork makes it both easy and exciting to learn. Breathing therapy truly works, and I tell everyone I know!

—Anjali Ranadive, Founder of Jaws and Paws

Nick is awesome! By learning self-awareness through his breathing exercises and environmental immersion, I've become more connected and grounded. Through my morning mindfulness routine, I've shifted toward a more positive and balanced lifestyle. Thank you, Nick Terry!

—Evan Walker, United Airlines Pilot

ABOUT THE AUTHOR

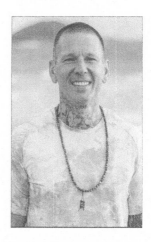

Nick Terry TNT is a certified life coach, certified breathwork practitioner, intervention consultant and an author. He is also the cofounder of Honu House Hawaii, a residential rehab facility in Kailua-Kona, Hawaii, and the owner of Breath of Life Recovery, a wellness consulting practice offering breathwork, cold water therapy and wellness modalities. Since getting sober in 2014, Nick has worked for more than eight years in the field of addiction and mental health treatment. He and his wife Paulina live with their two daughters Coco and Steisha in Maui, which he has called home for 22 years. *Breath of Life* is his first book.